beauty
superboosters

foods and massage to boost your natural beauty

amanda ursell

beauty
superboosters

foods and massage to boost your natural beauty

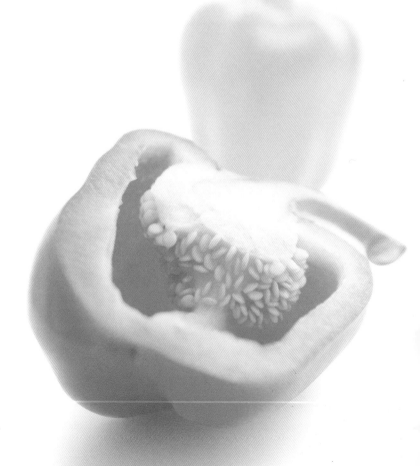

photography by russell sadur

For Bella, Emily, Fi and Hannah –
four of this world's natural beauties.

Beauty Superboosters
by Amanda Ursell

Beauty Superboosters is meant to be
used as a general reference and recipe
book. While the author believes the
information and recipes it contains are
beneficial to health, the book is in no
way intended to replace medical advice.
You are therefore urged to consult your
health-care professional about specific
medical issues or complaints.

First published in Great Britain in 2002
by Mitchell Beazley, an imprint of
Octopus Publishing Group Limited,
2–4 Heron Quays, London E14 4JP.
© Octopus Publishing Group
Limited 2002
Text © Amanda Ursell 2002

ISBN 1 84000 426 6

While all reasonable care has been
taken during the preparation of this
edition, neither the publisher, editors,
nor the author can accept responsibility
for any consequences arising from the
use thereof or from the information
contained therein.

Commissioning Editor: Rebecca Spry
Executive Art Editor: Phil Ormerod
Managing Editor: Jamie Grafton
Design: Nicky Collings
Editor: Jamie Ambrose
Production: Alix McCulloch,
Jessame Emms
Index: Laura Hicks
Special Photography: Russell Sadur
Author photograph on Jacket: Mike Prior

Typeset in Vectora
Printed and bound by
Toppan Printing Company in China

contents

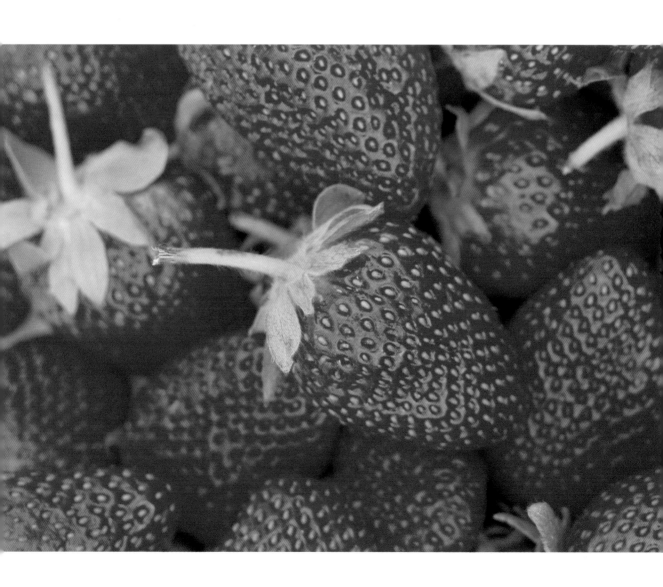

skin

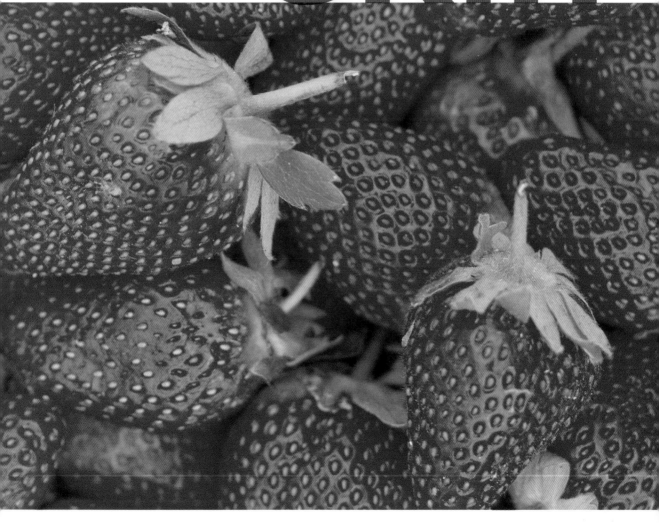

skin care

Skin is on show every day. How it looks can profoundly affect the way we feel about ourselves. If our skin looks good, we feel good, so it's little wonder that we spend so much time, effort, and money on beauty regimes. And so we should, because good-quality cleansing lotions and anti-ageing moisturizing creams applied to the surface of the skin are vital. Yet so, too, is a diet that not only takes into consideration the visible, very top layer of the skin, but also nourishes the layers of cells beneath it.

The epidermis is the part of the skin on show, made up of four to five layers of cells. The two outermost layers comprise dead, flattened cells, held together tightly by waterproofing fatty acids, oils, peptides, and ceramides – nature's way of creating a smooth barrier of moist, supple, and protective cells. In contrast, the three layers immediately beneath are very much alive: this is where the cells forming the skin we see are first manufactured. It is also where melanin – the pigment which determines skin colour and offers some protection against the destructive effects of the sun's ultraviolet radiation – is made. Some receptors involved in our sense of touch are also found here.

Under the epidermis lies the dermis – the corium or "true skin". It is a real hive of activity, packed with tiny arteries and veins, lymph vessels, and nerve fibres. Here, oil-producing glands are found, along with the roots of the fine hairs that cover the skin on your face and body. Oil glands and hair roots share the same blood supply, and the oil produced uses hair shafts as a route to the top skin layer, where it helps to retain moisture and keep the skin supple. The dermis is also home to sweat glands, which regulate temperature through perspiration, and detoxify the body by releasing some of the excess salt, ammonia, and other waste products of normal digestion and metabolism.

Crucially, the dermis also contains collagen and elastin: two structural proteins that act a bit like a body stocking, holding the body together. Collagen is made up from bundles of interlacing protein fibres, which tend to run lengthways in the skin of the head and neck, and in circular patterns around the neck and trunk. White in colour, collagen has a great ability to absorb shock, giving the skin strength and resilience and helping to keep it watertight. Elastin is also made from protein fibres, but while collagen absorbs knocks and physical stress, elastin is stretchy and springy. It gives the skin the ability to whiz back into shape after being pressed, pulled, or moved around – for example, when we tug it, smile, laugh, or make other facial expressions. In a nutshell, collagen gives the skin firmness, while its ability to return to its original shape is down to elastin.

The final layer of skin is fat, which (among other roles) helps to protect the body from physical knocks. This fat layer is found in even the slimmest people, although clearly it is much thicker when a person carries more weight. While the skin is the body's largest organ, the upper layers above the fat – where such a wide range of activities occur on a second-by-second basis – are no more than a fraction of a millimetre thick.

skin nourishment

To make radiant skin, the dermis must be supplied continually with oxygen, vitamins, minerals, essential fats, energy, and protein via tiny arteries. In addition, its network of little veins must remove carbon dioxide, along with other waste materials of metabolism. A hiccup in the supply of oxygen and nutrients or a long-term lack of either may reduce the speed of skin renewal and compromise both texture and condition.

skin colour

Skin colour is determined mainly by the pigment melanin, varying in colour from black to brown or yellow, made in special cells called melanocytes in the skin's epidermal layer. If melanocytes produce a lot of melanin, the skin is darker than when they make small amounts. In people of all colours, extra melanin is produced in the presence of sunlight, a mechanism that helps protect against the harmful effects of ultraviolet radiation. The reaction is more obvious in fair skin, where it results in a suntan. Freckles and moles are caused by localized build-ups of melanin. While melanin offers some protection against ultraviolet rays, excessive time outside can lead to burning and long-term damage of the skin's deeper layers, causing the clumping of elastin fibres, giving skin a leathery look. Two other pigments can influence the colour of skin. Betacarotene, the pigment found in carrots, sweet potatoes, and fruits such as peaches, apricots, and mangoes, can accumulate in the fatty layer of the skin, giving it an orange tinge, especially on the palms of the hands and soles of the feet. New research suggests it may actually offer some protection against sun damage. Meanwhile, haemoglobin, the red, oxygen-carrying component of blood, gives pale skin (which is actually almost transparent) its pinkish hue.

Emotions, of course, can also affect skin colour. Reddening or blushing can be caused by stress, while paleness can be stimulated through fear and anaemia. Both problems may be helped through diet. The blue-green effects of bruising are due to blood escaping from arteries and veins and clotting under the the skin's surface. Certain foods may strengthen blood-vessel walls and reduce the risk of bruising.

skin protection

As a physical barrier, skin helps prevent bacteria and other disease-causing agents from getting into the body. It also contains immune-system cells that help fight infections.

External stress on the skin, such as sunburn, can disrupt this immune protection, leading to (for example) the stimulation of the herpes virus and the appearance of cold sores.

nerves in the skin

The skin is home to millions of tiny receptors that feed information to the nerves and brain. If the body becomes too hot, sweat glands cause us to perspire, and the skin looks flushed. When you become too cold, blood vessels in the skin contract to stop heat loss, turning the skin pale and leaving it cold to the touch.

moisture

With the exception of the palms and soles of the feet, oil glands are found over all the skin's surface. They tend to be largest on the face, neck, and upper chest. The oil or "sebum" they produce slows water loss from the skin, and softens and lubricates both the skin and hair. It also seems to have some bacteria-fighting qualities. Oil production is controlled partly by hormones, which may be modified by the things we eat and drink.

skin facts

- The skin is the largest organ in the body.
- The human body is covered by approximately 1.5 to 2 square metres (2 to 2½ square yards) of skin, which weighs around 4kg (9 pounds).
- We rub off millions of dead skin cells every day and create a totally new top layer around every 40 days.
- 7 per cent of the average adult's body weight is made up of skin.
- Every square centimetre of skin contains an estimated 70cm (28 inches) of blood vessels, 55cm (22 inches) of nerves, 100 sweat glands, 15 oil glands, and 230 sense receptors.
- Skin varies in thickness from 1.5 to 4 millimetres ($1/_{16}$ to $1/_4$ inch) in different parts of the body.
- Few substances can enter the body via the skin. Exceptions include vitamins A, D, E, and K, and steroids.

skin
beauty foods

Other skin-softening foods

Mackerel, herring, sardines, flax seeds, chia seeds

salmon

promotes smooth, soft, watertight skin

what salmon does

Salmon may be useful in helping to keep skin **smooth**, **soft** in texture and **free from dry patches**, which can become itchy and red. Salmon and other oily fish may also **boost** the skin's **water-holding capacity**, giving it a **fresh**, plumped-up look. Well-hydrated skin tends to look **firmer** and be less prone to the development of fine lines and wrinkles.

why salmon works

Salmon is great for supplying the body with eicosapentanoic acid, or EPA, which is converted into specific hormone-like substances called prostaglandins. Prostaglandins are made by virtually every cell in the body, yet the prostaglandins produced from EPA have been found to restrict inflammation that could otherwise lead to dryness, which in turn can trigger itching and soreness. Salmon is also an excellent source of protein needed for the continuous production of collagen, keratin, and melanin, along with all other new and healthy skin cells.

salmon serving ideas

Salmon's meaty flesh makes it suitable for most methods of cooking. Salmon tastes good served hot or cold. Fresh salmon contains more EPA than smoked salmon.

salmon watchpoints

The farming of salmon has led to cheaper prices but also potential problems with pollution from rearing huge numbers of fish in confined spaces; occasionally, fish farms adopt poor practices involving contaminated feed. Although more expensive, organic salmon is thought to be safer for human consumption, and is undoubtedly better for the welfare of both fish and environment.

what watermelon does

Watermelon may help to keep the skin looking plump and **hydrated**, which in turn has the effect of **ironing out** some of the fine lines and making it **soft** to the touch. It may also play a role in keeping skin **supple** and **elastic**, helping to avoid the leathery, dry appearance of sun-damaged skin.

why watermelon works

One 200g (7oz) slice of watermelon provides as much fluid as a glass of water, so regular consumption can help reduce dehydration of the skin by replenishing part of the 500ml (18fl oz) of water it loses each day. This fruit's vibrant, red colour comes from a plentiful supply of carotene. Along with vitamin C, the carotene acts as an antioxidant, helping to neutralize free radicals generated by the sun's ultraviolet rays, which damage elastin and collagen and accelerate the process of skin ageing.

watermelon serving ideas

Wipe the dark-green skin with a clean cloth and cut into thick slices. Eat with your hands or cut into cubes and add to fruit salads or breakfast cereals. Watermelon can be puréed and made into sorbets, drinks, or summer soups. The skin can be carved into a melon basket and used to hold watermelon pieces and other mixed fruits.

watermelon watchpoints

Buy watermelons from stores that source this fruit from reputable growers. If grown in areas of polluted water, the fruit itself will take up and concentrate pollutants.

watermelon

helps hydrate skin and keep it supple

Other skin-hydrating foods

Ogen melon, yellow, red, and green peppers, lettuce, celery, cucumber

Other anti-ageing and circulation-boosting foods

Berries, oranges, kiwi fruit, spinach, peppers, sweet potatoes

papaya

anti-ageing and circulation-boosting

what papaya does

Papayas, also known as pawpaws, may help the skin **resist bruising** following minor knocks and bumps. Including papaya in the diet can help **bolster** the body's defences against sun exposure. This tropical fruit helps **boost** the skin's immune system and aids in the building, restoration, and maintenance of its **flexibility** and **youthful** appearance.

why papaya works

Papayas are rich in vitamin C and rutin, a plant nutrient that seems to help maintain the strength and stability of tiny blood vessels which are close to the skin's surface. A lack of vitamin C makes it easier for these walls to rupture when knocked, which in turn leads to bruising and tiny thread veins. Research suggests that large intakes of vitamin C, along with the orange betacarotene pigment found in papaya, may improve resistance to sunburn, bolster the effects of sunscreen products, and help in the renewal of collagen and elastin.

papaya serving ideas

Papayas can be cut in half lengthways and, once the seeds are removed, the flesh can be scooped out with a teaspoon. If peeled and cut into segments, the fruit can be served with lime and lemon juice or made into ice-cream. Papayas go well with pork, chicken, and scallops, and can be used in marinades to tenderize meat.

papaya watchpoints

The seeds taste peppery and hot, and while they may be puréed and added to salad dressings, they are not good when eaten raw. Fresh papaya contains an enzyme that will not allow gelatin to set, so avoid using it in jellies and mousse.

Other pollution-fighting foods

Fortified breakfast cereals, wholemeal bread, shellfish, wheat germ, sunflower seeds

brazil nuts

protect against free radicals, moisturize, and heal

what brazil nuts do

Brazil nuts may help **protect the skin** from the ageing effects of the sun's ultraviolet rays as well as from cigarette smoke in both active and passive smokers. They can also play a role in keeping the very top layers of skin **watertight** and the lower layers **moist** and **hydrated** to help reduce dryness. Brazil nuts may also be involved in reducing the problem of blemishes by promoting rapid **healing**.

why brazil nuts work

The selenium found in Brazil nuts is crucial for the production of the antioxidant glutathione peroxidase, which helps protect the skin from free-radical damage in the first twenty minutes of sun exposure. Combined with the vitamin E in Brazil nuts, selenium also helps neutralize free radicals in cigarette smoke, which trigger the release of collagen-attacking, skin-ageing MMP-1 enzymes. By zapping free radicals, glutathione peroxidase and vitamin E also help protect the skin's oil and essential fats that keep it watertight and hydrated, while vitamin E promotes skin healing.

brazil nut serving ideas

Chop and add to breakfast cereals such as muesli or porridge. When grated, Brazils can be mixed with cottage cheese and chopped peaches, or sprinkled over salads. Serve them whole with fruit and cheese. If blanched, chopped or grated, Brazils work witn bread mixes, nut burgers, and rissoles.

brazil nut watchpoints

The selenium content of Brazil nuts can range from 230 to 5,300 micrograms per 100g (3½oz). While it is essential to health, too much selenium is harmful, and intakes above 750 micrograms a day are inadvisable. People with nut allergies should, of course, avoid Brazil nuts.

what tofu does

It is suggested that tofu and other soya-based foods may be able to **slow** down some **age-related** changes in the skin, especially the rate of thinning and dryness that increases the speed at which lines and wrinkles develop. Tofu may also help in the general regeneration and **repair** of skin of all ages, and in maintaining a **strong**, **flexible** "mattress" of skin on which the upper layers rest.

why tofu works

Tofu and other soya-based foods such as milks and yoghurts contain plant nutrients known as isoflavones, specifically genistein, daidzein, and glycitein, which are similar in structure to the human hormone oestrogen. Oestrogen is needed to maintain the production of lubricating oils and good-quality collagen, which keep the skin moist, plump, and firm, and maintain its thickness. It is feasible that a diet rich in plant oestrogen may help counterbalance the reduction in human oestrogen as we age, and maintain a more youthful-looking skin.

tofu serving ideas

Tofu is the soft curd made from soya milk. Silken tofu has a soft and creamy texture and is great for making into dips, spreads, sauces, and puddings. It can be blended with fresh fruits such as bananas and strawberries to make a nutritious fruit smoothie, while the firmer version is ideal for stir-fries, sautéeing, and adding to casseroles or salads.

tofu watchpoints

The isoflavone content of tofu and other soya products varies widely, so it is usually not possible to determine daily intakes through food sources. Supplements offer an additional way of increasing plant-oestrogen intakes. Check labels carefully if you want to avoid genetically-modified soya.

tofu

aids collagen regeneration and anti-ageing

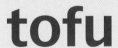

Other collagen-regenerating foods

Soya beans, soya milk, soya yoghurt, soya cheese, flax seeds

Other skin-revitalizing foods

Chamomile tea, lettuce, bananas, oats, St John's wort, kava kava

valerian

revitalizes tired skin and boosts tone

what valerian does

Valerian can help maximize the body's **regenerative** processes, potentially slowing the rate at which skin ages, and both creating and restoring a **healthy glow**. This distinctive-smelling herb could also reduce the appearance of dark circles under the eyes and play a role in keeping the skin **evenly coloured** and **clear**, with a good balance of oil and moisture.

why valerian works

Valerian contains substances called "valepotriates", which herbalists have long realized encourage a relaxed sleep. It is during the first cycle of sleep that our metabolism slows and the repair and renewal of cells can take place throughout the body – noticeably in the skin. A good night's sleep can reduce the development of dark circles under the eyes. Valerian's calming influence on the nervous system also reduces stress and the over-stimulation of oil glands, helping to keep skin colour and composition balanced.

valerian serving ideas

Soak 2 tsps of chopped fresh root in cold water for eight to ten hours, then drink in the evening with a little honey or peppermint water added to improve its somewhat earthy taste. Alternatively, take 5ml of valerian tincture a day, or 250 to 500mg in capsule or tablet form to help deal with stress.

valerian watchpoints

Do not use valerian drinks or tinctures while taking any medications prescribed to induce sleep, because this herb enhances their action. Take for two to three weeks, then take a break to avoid headaches.

Other moisturizing, skin-nourishing foods

Yoghurt, yoghurt drinks, calcium-enriched soya milk, mineral waters

milk

fosters plump, well-hydrated skin

what milk does

Milk helps maintain the continual **renewal of cells** in the skin and contributes to the daily **smooth growth** and **development** of skin structures, including the nerves that supply it. Milk can play a part in the regulation of water balance in the body, which is essential for the maintenance of **well-hydrated**, **firm-looking** skin.

why milk works

Milk is one of the richest suppliers of calcium, which is essential for the maturation and ongoing healthy growth and development of skin cells throughout the body. Magnesium, another essential mineral found in milk, is important for the smooth operation of nerves that supply the skin. A 200ml (7fl oz) glass of milk provides more than 175ml (6fl oz) of water, which helps boost fluid intake. Along with the potassium it contains, milk's water content contributes to good hydration.

milk serving ideas

Served chilled, skimmed milk can make a long, cool, refreshing drink. Add fresh fruits such as strawberries, bananas, and peaches, then blend to make nutritious smoothies and milk shakes. Warmed milk makes delicious, soothing hot chocolate and malted bedtime beverages. It can also be used both cold and hot on breakfast cereals or to make yoghurts, and may be added to soups to give body and nourishment .

milk watchpoints

Some people may be intolerant to milk and find that it aggravates dryness and eczema. Whole milk contains around 20g (almost 1oz) of fat per pint, compared to less than 1g in skimmed milk.

Other calming foods

Chamomile tea, lettuce, bananas, valerian, kava kava, St John's wort

oats

a de-stresser that reduces frown lines

what oats do

Oats may help to **reduce** the development of **frown lines** and wrinkles – especially those that form on the forehead and around the eyes. Regularly eating oats may also help **reduce thinning** of the skin, cutting down on the chances of broken veins and blemishes, and generally **slowing** the visible signs of **ageing**.

why oats work

Oats are known by herbalists to be an excellent nerve tonic, helping reduce the stress held around the body, including any in the face that can lead to the development of frown lines and stress wrinkles. Stress floods the body with hormones, thus increasing the heart rate, widening the blood vessels, and increasing the chances of flushing, hives, and broken veins. Stress can also over-stimulate sweat glands and increase the risk of spots. In addition to reducing these and other stress reactions, oats supply small amounts of silicon, which helps maintain collagen structure.

oat serving ideas

Cook oatmeal to make hot porridge or use raw to make muesli by mixing with nuts and dried fruits. Oats can be added to bread and malt loaves, or used in pancakes, muffins, and oatcakes. Herbalists make soothing drinks by simmering oat-straw and fresh oats in water.

oat watchpoints

Oats contain the protein gluten and should be avoided by those allergic to gluten or anyone suffering from coeliac disease.

what wholemeal bread does

Wholemeal bread can help maintain general **health** of the deeper, live skin layers, giving a **pinkish hue** to pale skin and maintaining **smoothness**. Regularly eating wholemeal bread may also **reduce** the appearance of **small broken veins** under the skin, as well as boosting its armoury of **antioxidant** nutrient stores, which may help maintain an even and **youthful** appearance.

why wholemeal bread works

Wholemeal bread supplies the body with iron, which is needed for the production of haemoglobin and the transportation of oxygen in the blood. It also provides good amounts of the B vitamin niacin, which helps prevent dryness. The fibre in wholemeal bread can cut the chances of constipation, which may otherwise raise blood pressure and can cause tiny ruptured thread veins in the face. Depending on its country of origin, the wheat in wholemeal bread can also be a rich source of selenium, zinc, and vitamin E. These fight free-radical damage from the sun's radiation, pollution, and smoke, potentially reducing the production of collagen-wrecking MMP-1 enzymes.

wholemeal bread serving ideas

Wholemeal bread is great with strong-flavoured cheese and pickles. Chunks of fresh wholemeal bread are excellent with filling soups and broths and as an alternative to potatoes with casseroles and stews.

wholemeal bread watchpoints

When eating a diet rich in fibre, it is essential to drink plenty of water. At least six to eight glasses are recommended daily. Water hydrates the fibre, which helps prevent constipation and eases the elimination of waste products.

wholemeal bread

boosts antioxidants to maintain youthful skin

Other antioxidant-boosting foods

Fortified breakfast cereals, brown rice, brown pasta, oats, rye bread

what wholegrain pasta does

Wholegrain pasta provides a steady supply of **energy** to all cells, including skin cells, thus helping to **fuel** and sustain the many metabolic processes continually at work in its **growth** and **maintenance**. It can also help **balance** the skin's metabolic processes and oil production.

why wholegrain pasta works

The slow drip-feeding of energy from wholegrain pasta to cells is due to the fact that it has a low glycaemic index and is broken down and digested slowly. Some herbalists and nutritionists believe that refined carbohydrates over-stimulate oil glands and increase the chances of oily skin. Wholegrain pasta also provides zinc, needed for strength of the dermis and for restoring an even appearance and texture to areas damaged by blemishes.

wholegrain pasta serving ideas

Wholegrain pasta's robust flavour needs a fairly strong-tasting sauce, with a style matched to the pasta's shape. Wholegrain spaghetti works well with a rich, tomato sauce, a macaroni dish requires a mature cheese in the sauce. Tasty served hot, wholegrain pasta shapes are also good cold in traditional pasta salads.

wholegrain pasta watchpoints

If wholegrain pasta's flavour is too strong, use half wholegrain and half white pasta. Wholegrain pasta contains large amounts of dietary fibre, so drink water with meals to reduce the risk of indigestion.

wholegrain pasta

provides slow-release energy for skin cells

Other energy foods

Fortified wheat flakes, oats

Other healing foods

Fortified wheat flakes and breakfast wheat biscuits, wholemeal bread, shellfish, red meat

bran flakes

nourish and heal skin

what bran flakes do

This breakfast cereal can contribute to a glowing, **radiant** skin, which is well-moisturized, smooth, and **nourished**. Bran flakes may be particularly useful for maintaining the condition of skin that is regularly exposed to sunlight, and for helping in the **healing** of blemishes, scratches, and small wounds. Regular intakes may also help the skin **fight infections**.

why bran flakes work

Bran flakes are generally fortified with a range of vitamins and minerals, including iron, which is essential for carrying oxygen-rich blood to the tiny arteries supplying and feeding the skin. This helps to maximize growth and development of new cells deep within the dermis. It also allows for the upkeep and regeneration of structures within the skin, such as hair follicles and oil glands. The B vitamin niacin in bran flakes helps protect skin exposed to sunlight, while zinc is crucial for healing and a healthy immune system.

bran flake serving ideas

Bran flakes can be served alone with fresh, cool milk or with extra fruit. Grated apple and chopped banana make ideal partners. The flakes also go well with sultanas, raisins, and nuts, creating a tasty "fruit-and-fibre" mix.

bran flake watchpoints

Bran flakes are a rich source of dietary fibre. When increasing fibre intakes, it is important at the same time to increase fluid intake in order to avoid constipation.

Other skin-renewing foods

Haddock, red and grey mullet, whiting, cod, mussels

seaweed

for constant skin renewal

what seaweed does

The chances of developing a **smooth** and **flexible** skin may be enhanced if seaweed is included in meals. It can help keep the cells of the dermis growing at a regular, normal rate. Seaweed may also contribute to maintaining the skin's **firmness** and **elasticity**, to help reduce the risk of fine lines and promote rapid **healing** when the skin is damaged.

why seaweed works

Seaweed is a great source of iodine, which, when in short supply, can slow the growth of skin and leave it dry and scaly by compromising the function of the thyroid gland. Many seaweeds are also rich in copper, a nutrient crucial for the formation of cross-links in collagen (which gives skin strength and springiness) and for extra elasticity in elastin. Seaweed provides the dermal layers of the skin with zinc, which helps repair skin cells damaged through cuts and grazes.

seaweed serving ideas

Kombu – wide-leafed, ribbon-like seaweed – is a greenish colour and is used to add flavour to stocks and soups; when dried, it can be crumbled over rice. Nori is available in flat sheets; again, it's added to soups and stews and is used to wrap sushi. Wakame, a deep-green, curly-leafed seaweed, is used in salads and soups.

seaweed watchpoints

Buy from reputable sources which are guaranteed to have been grown in unpolluted waters. Store dried seaweed away from damp places.

what prawns do

Prawns can play a role in helping the skin maintain optimal production of its **springy** underlying mattress. This gives the skin an impression of **firmness**, and helps collagen spring back into place following normal facial movements. Prawns may also assist the skin in the creation of its **natural protection against ultraviolet radiation**, and in maintaining even skin **tone** and **colour**.

why prawns work

Copper, found in prawns, is a key trace element in the formation of melanin, the pigment that helps absorb ultraviolet rays and creates a consistent, natural skin colour. It is also crucial for the formation of one of the body's most potent antioxidants, an anti-ageing enzyme called superoxide dismutase. In addition, the copper in prawns is a vital building-block for both cushioning collagen and springy elastin, which develop in the deeper skin layers.

prawn serving ideas

Prawns are particularly suited to grilling, barbecuing, and pan- or stir-frying. Serve them whole with the shell in dishes such as paella, or use the meaty tail in salads, on kebabs alternated with peppers and other vegetables, in curries, stir-fries, or in mixed seafood dishes. Prawns are particularly suited to Oriental and Asian cooking.

prawn watchpoints

Most prawns consumed are frozen, so always store them according to instructions and use before the use-by date to avoid any risk of food-poisoning. Avoid prawns with loose heads and black legs; this indicates bad condition.

prawns

help even skin colour, tone, and texture

Other texture-promoting foods

Seafood, wholegrains, pulses, nuts, liver

what sweet potatoes do

Eating sweet potatoes regularly may help **protect** the skin from the immediate burning and redness caused by exposure to the sun's ultraviolet rays. They may also help maintain **moisture** and **texture** and reduce the risk of wrinkles and lines after longer-term exposure, as well as playing a role in allowing **recovery** from **sun damage** to take place.

why sweet potatoes work

Sweet potatoes are rich in three powerful antioxidants: betacarotene and vitamins E and C. When it accumulates in the skin, betacarotene seems to diffuse the sun's ultraviolet rays. This, in turn, appears to enhance protection from externally applied UV-protecting sun creams, lessening the immediate burning effect on the skin. All of these antioxidants may help reduce the release of the sun-induced, collagen-damaging MMP-1 enzyme. Vitamin C can also assist in collagen repair, while vitamin E helps repair superficial damage.

sweet potato serving ideas

Sweet potatoes can be baked in their skins and served like jacket potatoes as a vegetable with a main meal or as a dish in their own right with cheese, chilli, or other savoury fillings. They can be cut into thick wedges for roasting, and their sweet flavour makes them ideal for mashing. Add to casseroles and stews, or purée and use in savoury soufflés.

sweet potato watchpoints

Be sure to buy red sweet potatoes, which have an orange-coloured flesh, since white versions are not as rich in betacarotene. Scrub and wash skins well to remove dirt before use.

sweet potatoes

protect against ultraviolet radiation

Other skin-protection foods

Carrots, spinach, kale, papayas, mangoes, apricots, peaches

strawberries

protect the skin's collagen and elastin structure

what strawberries do

Strawberries may help reduce the skin's loss of elasticity and firmness as we age by **protecting its collagen and elastin structure**. Regular consumption may **lower the risk** of bruising and of the tiny thread veins that appear just under the skin's surface. Strawberries are one of the few fruits potentially capable of **combating** the negative effects of smoking and modern **pollutants** in our bodies.

Other structure-protecting foods

Blueberries, oranges, kiwi fruit, red and green peppers, spinach

why strawberries work

Strawberries are rich in vitamin C and bioflavonoids, two nutrients that are crucial for maintaining strong capillary walls. Strong walls protect against rupturing, and thus unsightly bruising and thread veins. Strong capillaries also ensure a constant and effective supply of oxygen and nutrients to elastin and collagen in the skin, which allow its continual regeneration. Strawberries are packed with ellagic acid, which helps destroy the hydrocarbons in cigarette smoke that are capable of damaging the lungs and the skin.

strawberry serving ideas

Serve whole in a bowl, with or without a creamy topping such as fromage frais or yoghurt. Sprinkle with a little caster sugar or a drizzle of white wine or lemon or orange juice. Fresh and frozen strawberries are both ideal for combining with bananas to create a delicious smoothie or to make cool sorbets and summer-fruit soups.

strawberry watchpoints

Always wash strawberries to rinse off residual dirt and pesticides. Although rare, some people experience an allergic rash after eating strawberries.

**Other
anti-thinning foods**
Oats, muesli, oat-straw

horsetail

maintains skin thickness

what horsetail does

Horsetail is a herb that may help **reduce** the natural **thinning** of skin, which occurs gradually from the late-20s onwards. It even has the potential to **restore** the thickness of the upper and lower layers of the skin as we age. Horsetail is also said to **improve** areas of dryness and elevate **moisture** levels, effects which could combine to reduce the appearance of fine lines.

why horsetail works

Horsetail is one of the few good suppliers of silicon, considered a trace element by some practitioners. The highest concentrations of silicon in the human body are found in the skin, indicating its importance to this organ. Used by herbalists to beautify skin, silicon seems to maintain the amorphous material between collagen and elastin fibres which helps prevent the thickening and tangling that leads to the thinning and ageing of the skin. Early research suggests that good intakes of silicon may both protect against and reverse signs of skin ageing.

horsetail serving ideas

The fresh, aerial parts of the horsetail herb resemble thyme in appearance and can be made into a drink by simmering 25g (1oz) dried or 55g (2oz) fresh plant in 750ml (26fl oz) of water for an hour, or until it reduces to 500ml (18fl oz). Sip one cup of this "tea" three times a day. Juice can also be made by liquidizing the stems, and 5ml to 10ml (1 to 2 tsp) can be drunk daily. Alternatively, horsetail can be taken in capsule form, following dosage instructions on the packet.

horsetail watchpoints

If, on taking horsetail, menstrual flow becomes heavier than normal, seek help from a qualified medical herbalist.

what evening primrose oil does

Fine lines and **wrinkles** may seem less apparent when regularly taking evening primrose oil, and the skin can take on a **smoother texture** after a few months of including this oil in the diet. The oil has been known to **heal small scars** left after spots, scratches, and **blemishes**, and has been shown to counteract dryness and even heal red, itchy patches.

why evening primrose oil works

Evening primrose oil is a source of the essential fat known as linoleic acid, which is crucial for keeping skin cells watertight and for retaining moisture levels, thus maintaining a plump appearance. In addition, it is one of the few sources of gamma linolenic acid, or GLA. GLA is converted in the body into certain hormone-like substances called prostaglandins, which play a part in controlling the quantity of oil secreted, and can reduce inflammation, and thus redness and itching.

evening primrose oil serving ideas

Evening primrose oil can be bought in capsules or in small dropper bottles. Capsules can be made from gelatin or a vegetarian material. The oil from dropper bottles can be taken on a spoon or added to food. Its slightly nutty flavour goes well in soups or cereals; you could even try dropping it onto slices of toast.

evening primrose oil watchpoints

It is crucial to buy a good-quality oil with guaranteed levels of at least ten per cent GLA. For any noticeable effects, at least four to six 500mg capsules need to be taken daily for at least four weeks.

evening primrose oil

promotes moist, smooth, soft skin

Other skin-smoothing foods

Blackcurrant oil, flax seeds, pumpkin seeds, sesame seeds, sunflower seeds

7–day skin diet

	breakfast	lunch	dinner
1	strawberry smoothie	mozzarella and plum tomato salad	marinated tofu and tamari salad with mint
2	bircher-style muesli with raspberries	butter bean hummus with fresh mint and toast	tuna steak with new potato salad
3	salmon bagel	cashew nut rice salad with mango	tandoori chicken with basmati rice
4	brazil nut and peach bran flakes	sweet-potato soup	pancake with prawns and salad
5	papaya and lime fruit salad	prawn and vermicelli soup	beef shallots with Dijon mustard mash
6	wake-up shake	salmon and fennel on rye	tofu and chilli stir-fry with bean sprouts
7	granary to go	penne salad with chicken and lemon	stir-fry prawns with watercress and sesame

day 1 *recipes*

strawberry smoothie

100g (3½oz) fresh or frozen strawberries

1 small banana, peeled

1 small pot plain bio-yoghurt

150ml (5fl oz) skimmed milk or soya milk

crushed ice, to serve

Place all ingredients in a blender. Blend well and serve over crushed ice in a glass.

mozzarella and plum tomato salad

2 slices rye bread, cut into croûtons

1 garlic clove, crushed

salt and freshly ground black pepper

extra-virgin olive oil

3 ripe plum tomatoes

55g (2oz) mozzarella

1 tsp balsamic vinegar

a few fresh basil leaves, torn

fat-free vinaigrette dressing

1 handful prepared salad leaves

1. Pre-heat the grill to maximum. Place the croûtons on a baking tray and mix in the crushed garlic. Season with a little salt and freshly ground black pepper, then drizzle with a little oil. Place under the grill to crisp.
2. Slice the tomatoes and mozzarella, and lay on a heatproof serving plate in alternate layers. Sprinkle with freshly ground pepper.
3. Remove the toasted rye croûtons from the heat, then warm the mozzarella and tomatoes under the grill for a minute or two. Remove from the grill and drizzle with balsamic vinegar. Garnish with a few torn leaves of fresh basil.
4. Add the fat-free dressing to the salad leaves and then sprinkle with the toasted rye bread croûtons. Serve with the mozzarella and tomatoes.

marinated tofu and tamari salad with mint

100g (3½oz) egg noodles

2 tbsps soy sauce

juice of 1 lemon

a small piece of fresh ginger, finely grated

a few fresh mint leaves, chopped

1 tsp runny honey

85g (3oz) marinated or smoked tofu

100g (3½oz) fresh bean sprouts

2 tomatoes, chopped

2 spring onions

1. Cook the egg noodles as per the instructions on the packet. Meanwhile, put the soy sauce, lemon juice, grated ginger, mint, and honey into a large bowl, whisk well, and leave to marinate.
2. Cut the tofu into dice-size pieces and then warm it through, either in a steamer or in a sieve over the pan of boiling noodles.
3. Add the bean sprouts to the soy sauce mixture and mix well. Drain the noodles, then add to the mixture with the tomatoes and spring onion, and mix thoroughly. Add the tofu, saving a few pieces for presentation, and drizzle with any remaining dressing.

day 2 *recipes*

bircher-style muesli with raspberries

2 tbsps skimmed milk

15g (½oz) rolled oat flakes

1 tsp oatmeal

55g (2oz) plain fromage frais

1 tsp runny honey

1 small apple

100g (3½oz) fresh or frozen raspberries

1 tsp honey-roast sunflower seeds

1. Warm the milk. Pour over the oats and oatmeal, and leave to soak overnight in the fridge.
2. When ready to eat, stir in the fromage frais and honey. Grate the apple and mix in, along with half the raspberries. Use the rest to top the muesli and sprinkle with the sunflower seeds.

butter bean hummus with fresh mint and toast

55g (2oz) cooked or canned butter beans

1 tbsp virtually fat-free plain fromage frais

1 tsp crunchy peanut butter

1 drop Tabasco sauce

a few fresh mint leaves, chopped

salt & freshly ground black pepper

pinch of curry powder

2 slices wholemeal bread

1 medium carrot, peeled

1 stick celery

half a cucumber

1. Place the butter beans in a small blender and add the fromage frais, peanut butter, Tabasco, mint, a tiny pinch of salt (leave this out if using canned beans), pepper, and curry powder. Blend until smooth, then taste for seasoning. Spice up with more Tabasco if needed.
2. Toast the bread. Cut the vegetables into suitably sized sticks for dipping into the butter-bean hummus. Spread a little hummus on the toast, and serve the rest as a dip for the vegetable sticks.

tuna steak with new potato salad

Extra-virgin olive oil

100g (3½oz) fresh tuna steak

Salt & freshly ground black pepper

200g (7oz) cooked new potatoes, cold

1 tsp grain mustard

1 small bunch chives, chopped

1 spring onion, finely chopped

1 tbsp fat-free salad dressing

Juice of half a lime

1 ripe plum tomato, sliced

A small cos lettuce (or baby gem)

1. Brush a non-stick frying pan lightly with olive oil; pre-heat. Season the tuna steak with a little salt and lots of pepper; place in the pan to cook gently for two minutes on each side.
2. To make the potato salad: slice the cooked potatoes in half, then mix in the grain mustard, chives, spring onion, and salad dressing. Mix the salad with a fork.
3. When the tuna has cooked, remove from the pan and sprinkle with the lime juice. Leave to rest for a few moments. Serve on the plum tomato slices and lettuce, with the new potato salad on the side.

day 3 *recipes*

salmon bagel

1 bagel

2 tsps reduced-fat
cream cheese

25g (1oz) smoked salmon

juice of ½ lemon

freshly ground black pepper

1. Slice the bagel in half and spread each side with the cream cheese.
2. Divide the salmon between the halves; lay over the cheese, sprinkle with lemon juice, and top with ground black pepper.

cashew nut rice salad with mango

15g (½oz) salted cashew nuts,
roughly chopped
½ fresh mango,
peeled and cubed

½ red pepper,
de-seeded and chopped

4 heaped tbsps cooked brown rice

1 tbsp chopped chives

1 small bunch spring onions,
finely chopped

1 tbsp chopped parsley

salt and freshly ground
black pepper

lettuce leaves

juice of ½ lemon

1. Heat a small frying pan and add the nuts, cooking gently to release their flavour.
2. Mix the mango with the pepper and rice. Add the chives, spring onions, lemon juice, and parsley.
3. Once the nuts are lightly toasted, mix half into the salad. Season to taste, place in a bowl on top of some lettuce leaves, and sprinkle with the remaining nuts.

tandoori chicken with basmati rice

1 tsp tandoori seasoning

55g (2oz) virtually fat-free
set yoghurt

100g (3½oz) skinless chicken breast

salt and freshly ground black pepper

½ garlic clove, crushed

juice of ½ lemon

4 level tbsps basmati rice, soaked
in cold water

pinch of turmeric

300ml (10fl oz) vegetable stock

55g (2oz) sultanas

mixed salad leaves, to serve

1. Mix the tandoori seasoning with the yoghurt. Season the chicken with salt and pepper, then rub with garlic, lemon juice, and the tandoori yoghurt. Grill for five to six minutes each side.
2. Drain the rice. Put into a pan with the turmeric, sultanas, vegetable stock, and a tiny pinch of salt. Bring to the boil and leave to cook for three to four minutes. Cover with a tight-fitting lid, then turn off the heat.
3. Remove the chicken from heat and leave to rest, then slice into thin strips. Place the strips and cooking juices on the leaves; serve with rice.

day 4 *recipes*

brazil nut and peach bran flakes

40g (1½oz) bran flakes

1 fresh peach, stoned and sliced

skimmed milk

2 Brazil nuts, shelled and finely chopped

1. Put the bran flakes into a bowl; add the peach slices and milk.
2. Sprinkle with the nuts and serve.

sweet-potato soup

extra-virgin olive oil

½ medium onion, peeled and finely chopped

100g (3½oz) orange sweet potato, peeled and finely diced

½ red chilli, chopped

1 garlic clove, crushed

1 tsp tomato purée

1 tsp mild curry paste

1 tbsp crunchy peanut butter

700ml (25fl oz) vegetable stock (use an organic stock cube)

1 standard can chopped tomatoes

1 large tbsp plain fromage frais

freshly ground black pepper

chilli sauce (optional)

1. In a medium-sized pan brushed lightly with oil, cook the onion and sweet potato for three to four minutes, stirring continuously, until softened.
2. Add the chilli, garlic, tomato purée, and curry paste, and continue to cook for three to four minutes more. Add the peanut butter, vegetable stock, and canned tomatoes. Bring to the boil, then turn down the heat and simmer for 12 to 15 minutes, until the vegetables are soft.
3. Remove from heat, then pour into a food processor or liquidizer and blend until smooth. Serve with a good spoonful of fromage frais. Adjust the seasoning with black pepper and add a little chilli sauce if you like your soup with more spice. This soup freezes well and will improve in flavour if allowed to rest for a day.

pancake with prawns and salad

25g (1oz) buckwheat flour

25g (1oz) plain flour

100ml (3½fl oz) skimmed milk

1 egg white

salt and freshly ground black pepper

2 tbsps extra-virgin olive oil

55g (2oz) cooked, peeled prawns

juice of ½ lemon

a small piece cucumber, chopped

2 ripe plum tomatoes, chopped

mixed salad leaves

1. Beat together the buckwheat, plain flour, milk, and egg white, along with a tiny pinch of salt. If the mixture is lumpy, pass it through a sieve. Lightly coat a non-stick frying pan with the oil, and heat. Add enough batter to cover the base of the pan. Cook for about two minutes, then gently turn the pancake over to cook the other side for one minute only.
2. Season the prawns with lemon juice and black pepper, then mix with the cucumber and tomatoes.
3. When the pancake is done, transfer to a plate. Place the prawn mixture and mixed salad leaves on one side of the pancake. Fold over to serve.

day 5 *recipes*

papaya and lime fruit salad

½ small papaya, peeled, de-seeded and sliced

1 orange, peeled and cut into segments

juice of 1 fresh lime

1 tbsp low-fat Greek yoghurt

Mix the fruits together and squeeze over the fresh lime juice. Top with the yoghurt and serve.

prawn and vermicelli soup

1 vegetable or chicken stock cube (use an organic stock cube)

500ml (18fl oz) boiling water

2 spring onions, chopped

1 tbsp teriyaki sauce

55g (2oz) wholegrain vermicelli

zest of half a lemon

100g (3½oz) cooked prawns

fresh coriander leaves, chopped, for garnish

1 salad or plum tomato, chopped, for garnish

1 large slice rye bread, warmed

1. Dilute the stock cube in water, pour into a suitable pan and heat to simmering. Add the spring onions, and teriyaki sauce.

2. Pour boiling water onto the vermicelli, enough to completely cover it. After a few minutes, drain and add to the stock.

3. Now add the lemon zest and prawns, being careful not to boil, or else the prawns will overcook. Remove from heat.

4. To serve, garnish with a little freshly chopped coriander and chopped tomato for colour. Serve immediately with a slice of warmed rye bread.

beef shallots with Dijon mustard mash

200g (7oz) potatoes, peeled and chopped

70g (2½oz) organic sirloin fillet

salt and freshly ground black pepper

2 tsps Dijon mustard

1 shallot, peeled and finely chopped

mixture of baby vegetables: carrots, sweetcorn, and mange-tout

grated nutmeg

100ml (3½fl oz) skimmed milk

1. Cook the potatoes in salty water until soft.

2. Meanwhile, cover the beef in a sheet of clingfilm and flatten it with a rolling pin or the base of a pan. Season, then spread a tsp of Dijon mustard on one side and sprinkle with the chopped shallot. Grill, shallot-side up, on a suitable baking sheet for four to five minutes.

3. Steam the baby vegetables. Once the potatoes are ready, drain, then return to the pan. Add a little grated nutmeg, the milk, and a tsp of Dijon mustard. Mash the potatoes well until smooth.

4. Serve the mustard mash and steak with the baby vegetables on the side.

day 6 *recipes*

wake-up shake

4 kiwi fruits, peeled and chopped
50ml (2fl oz) orange juice
150ml (5fl oz) plain low-fat yoghurt
1 ripe banana, peeled
1 tbsp ice-cubes, crushed
fresh mint, for garnish

Put all ingredients into a blender and whiz until smooth. Pour into a chilled glass and serve garnished with mint.

salmon and fennel on rye

½ bulb of fennel
55g (2oz) canned red salmon, drained
1 tsp horseradish
1 tsp fresh lemon juice
1 tbsp plain fromage frais
2 tsps freshly chopped chives
pinch of salt
freshly ground black pepper
2 slices rye bread or 4 rye crispbreads
1 handful mixed salad leaves

1. Grate the fennel coarsely into a bowl and add the salmon. Mix well with a fork.
2. Add all the remaining ingredients (apart fropm the bread and salad), reserving some chopped chives for garnish, and stir thoroughly.
3. Spread over the bread or crispbreads, garnish with the reserved chives, and serve with the salad leaves.

tofu and chilli stir-fry with bean sprouts

100g (3½oz) plain or marinated tofu
sesame oil
2 spring onions, finely sliced
1 red pepper, finely chopped
1 yellow pepper, finely chopped
1 carrot, peeled and grated
100g (3½oz) bean sprouts
1 red chilli, finely chopped with a little white sugar (to reduce heat)
2 tbsps teriyaki sauce
2 tsps fish sauce
200g (7oz) rice noodles (cooked weight)
1 small bunch fresh coriander, chopped

1. Bring a pan of salty water to the boil, ready to re-heat the rice noodles. Cut the tofu into small cubes and stir-fry in the oil for a couple of minutes.
2. Add the spring onions, de-seeded peppers, grated carrot, and the bean sprouts. Add the chilli. Toss well.
3. Add the teriyaki and fish sauces.
4. Re-heat the noodles in the boiling water; drain in a colander or sieve.
5. Arrange the stir-fry on top of the noodles to serve. Garnish with some freshly chopped coriander.

day 7 *recipes*

granary to go

2 slices granary bread
peanut butter
1 small apple

Toast the granary bread and spread with peanut butter. Grate the apple and pile on top. Make a sandwich and enjoy!

penne salad with chicken and lemon

115g (4oz) cooked wholegrain penne
1 tsp Dijon mustard
2 tsps lemon juice
1 tsp tomato purée
1 tbsp low-fat Greek yoghurt
few drops Tabasco sauce
pinch of sugar
salt and freshly ground black pepper
¼ cucumber, diced
1 ripe tomato, diced
100g (3½oz) cooked chicken, chopped
1 tbsp chopped chives

1. Cook the pasta according to the packet instructions, drain and cool.
2. In a bowl, mix together the mustard, lemon juice, tomato purée, yoghurt, Tabasco, sugar, and a little salt and pepper to season. Add the cucumber and tomato, chicken, and chives.
3. Mix well with the pasta. Sprinkle with more pepper and serve.

stir-fry prawns with watercress and sesame

14 raw shelled tiger prawns
80g (2¾oz)sesame seeds
2 egg whites mixed with 2 tsp cornflour
1 tablespoon sunflower oil
2 cloves crushed garlic
a bunch of watercress leaves
100g (3½oz)beansprouts
100g (3½oz)cooked rice noodles
4 carrots peeled and grated
1 tablespoon light soy a sauce
1 tablespoon fish sauce
a bunch of fresh coriander

1. Heat a little oil in a wok. Season the prawns with a little salt and pepper and roll in the egg white and cornflour and in the sesame seeds.
2. Fry the prawns lightly for 3–4 minutes, then rest on a warm plate.
3. Heat a little more oil, then add the the onions, beansprouts, garlic, carrots, then finally the watercress.
4. Once the vegetables are cooking add the cooked rice noodles with the soya sauce and Thai fish sauce.
5. Turn the stirfry out onto a plate, place the prawns around and sprinkle with freshly chopped coriander.

skin
beauty massage

Around thirty muscles are responsible for facial expressions. When you are stressed, it shows on your face in the form of a worried, pinched look; over time, these "frown lines" become etched in the expression. Regularly massaging your face stimulates and relaxes the sensory nerves and complex muscles in your neck, face, forehead, and scalp. It also helps stimulate the circulation, thus bringing more oxygen and nutrients to muscles, which helps keep the skin toned, the complexion fresh, and you looking younger. Try to give yourself a complete facial massage once or twice a week.

complexion brightener

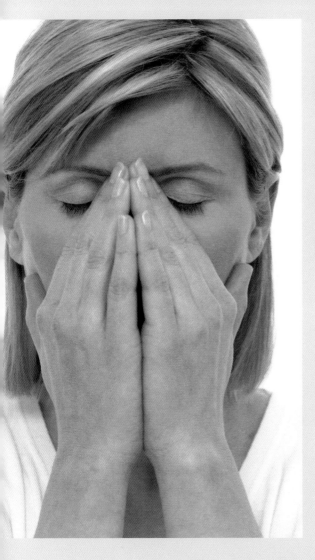

Place the palms of your hands on your jawline so that your fingertips rest lightly on your cheekbones, and pause for a moment. With light, even pressure, glide three fingers in a sweeping movement up either side of your nose, through the middle of your forehead, and down along your hairline.

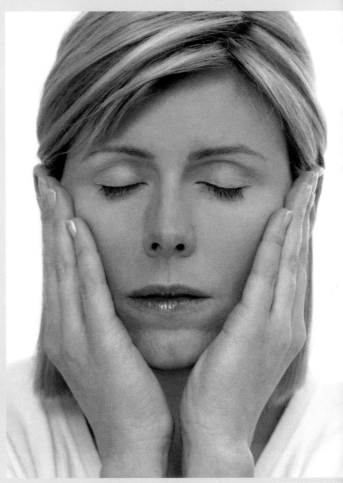

Continue down the temples to join at the middle of your jaw. Repeat five times.

smooth away frown lines, part 1

1 Place the pads of three fingers of both hands at the bridge of your nose between the eyebrows (this is an important acupressure point).

2 Hold the pressure there for a few seconds, then make small circular movements outward across your forehead toward the temples. Repeat three times.

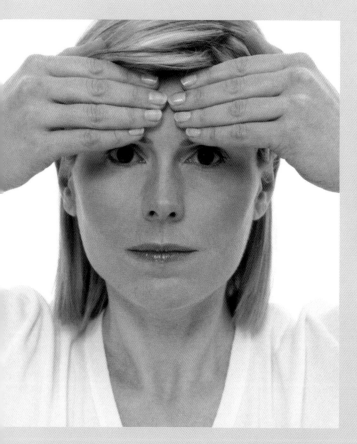
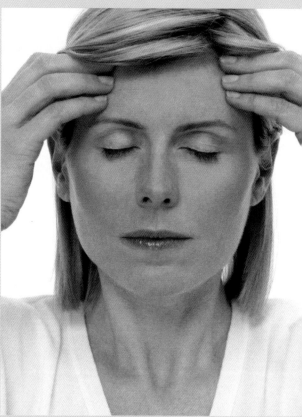

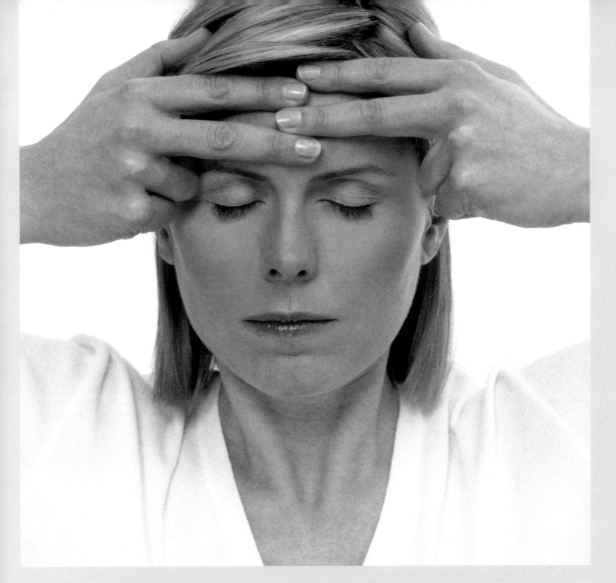

smooth away frown lines, part 2

1 Form the index and middle fingers of both hands into a horizontal "v" across your forehead and gently rub them in a scissor-like action across the middle of the forehead, above the eyebrows, and out toward the temples. Repeat three times.

deep tension release

With the pads of your fingers, start at the bridge of your nose and make circular movements in a straight line up your forehead to your hairline.

Thoroughly work the whole head with firm, circular pressure all over the scalp, as if shampooing your hair. Concentrate on moving the skin of the scalp rather than moving the hair.

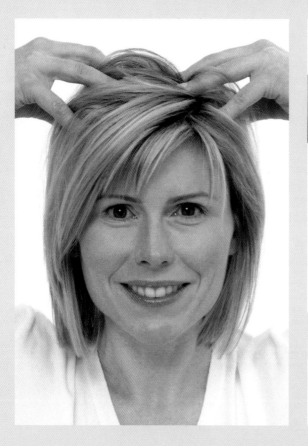
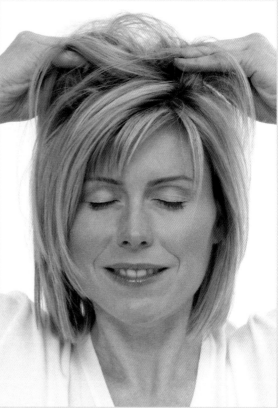

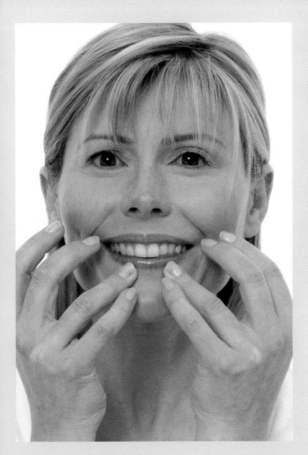

face reviver

Using your fingertips, lightly tap with a feathery touch all over your face, starting with your chin and working out toward your jaw. Move up and feather-touch across the cheeks to your ears, then from your forehead out toward your temples.

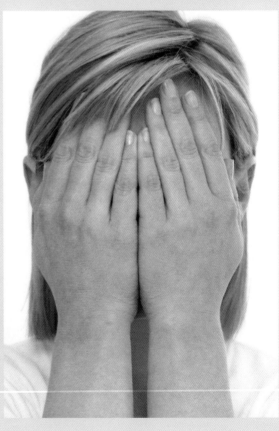

Finish your skin massage by cupping both hands over your face. Hold for a few moments to feel the heat from your hands. Slowly release, gliding your hands out toward the temples; feather-touch across the cheeks to your ears, then from your forehead out toward your temples.

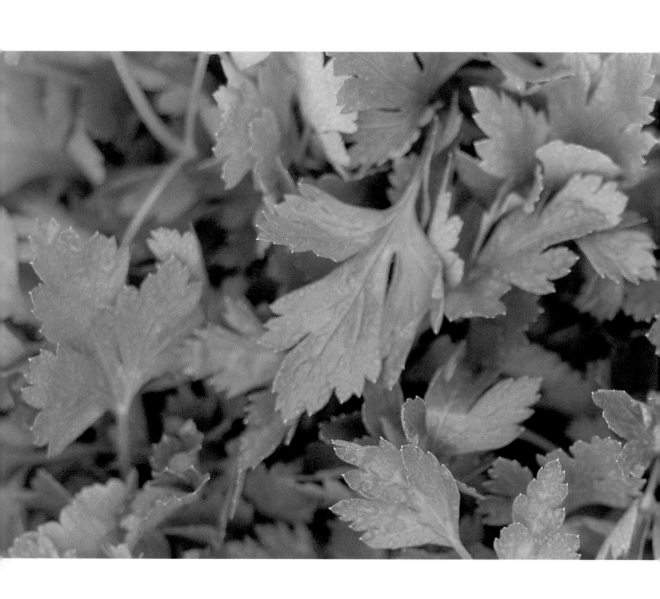

mouth

mouth care

Kissable lips and sweet-smelling breath are not simply the results of lipstick and peppermints. A beautiful mouth also needs care and nurturing from the inside out.

lickable lips

Seductive, sensuous, and soft, lips are actually fleshy types of muscle; the upper-lip muscle starts at the base of the nose, and the lower-lip muscle reaches down to the chin. The parts we think of as the lips are translucent areas of skin that allow the blood in the underlying capillaries to show through. The red margin of the lips contains no sweat or oil glands, which is why lips tend to become dry and cracked, and why we naturally moisten them by frequently licking them. The edges of the red margin are particularly prone to drying and cracking. While this may be caused through the heat, cold, or wind, a lack of certain nutrients can also be to blame, and this can be helped through diet.

lip lines

Fine, feathery lines appear around the lips as we age. While difficult to avoid, good circulation and plenty of collagen-boosting nutrients may help keep them at bay.

If more permanent-looking lines have started to appear around the mouth, then it is never too late to work on your expressions. Smile more, move the muscles, and start now with a regular massage routine.

terrific teeth

As soon as you smile and speak, the lips draw back and your teeth are on display. While their obvious role is to chew food, maintaining great-looking teeth and a Julia Roberts smile is part of any serious beauty regime. You do not need to live with crooked, discoloured teeth – these problems can be corrected by professional treatment – yet healthy gums and teeth are both areas for which you are largely responsible.

Teeth are made up of two main sections: the crown, which is the part you see, covered with familiar white enamel, and the root, which lies hidden below the gums. Enamel is the hardest substance in the body and is made mostly of calcified salts. A bone-like substance called dentine lies under the enamel, and beneath this is a soft material, the pulp, which contains the blood vessels and nerves that supply the tooth with nutrients and sensitivity. Cavities occur when the hard enamel of the tooth is damaged. This damage can be reduced by minimizing plaque, a film of sugar, bacteria, and other mouth debris that sticks to the teeth. Plaque creates acid that dissolves the calcified salts in enamel. Gums can also be badly affected by plaque, and healthy gums are crucial for maintaining a fresh, good-looking mouth. When plaque builds up where the tooth meets the gum, it leads to the build-up of tartar which, in turn, sets up infections, causing redness, soreness, and swollen, bleeding gums. These periodontal problems lead to considerable discomfort and stress, which are quickly translated into having little to smile about. Inflammation of the gums is known as gingivitis; this, at its worst, can lead to a disease called pyorrhea, a problem that accounts for eight per cent of tooth loss in adults and the unsightly development of receding gums.

Brushing and flossing are crucial for a fabulous mouth, but what and when you eat can drastically reduce the chances of tooth decay and gum disease, helping you to keep that fantastic smile for years to come.

erosion

A relatively new problem is the wearing away of teeth due to chemical erosion, in which acids contained in foods soften the enamel, which is then literally spat down the sink when brushing. Although citrus fruits and juices are full of nutrients beneficial to the mouth, they also contain citric acid, which contributes to this erosive effect. Eating and drinking fruits and fruit juices at mealtimes, rather than on their own, helps diminish their erosive capabilities. The same is true for vinegar (which contains acetic acid), apples (which contain malic acid), and rhubarb (which contains oxalic acid). Cola drinks are packed with phosphoric acid, so if it's a fabulous mouth you are seeking, the best advice is to give these teeth-eroding drinks a miss.

saliva

A good flow of saliva helps to cleanse the mouth between meals, flushing away some of the bacteria that can otherwise lead to bad breath and tooth decay. A lack of saliva can also lead to dry, cracked lips. Keeping up your fluids is vital for regular saliva production; waiting until you are thirsty is too late. By this time, the body is already dehydrated, so get used to increasing your water intake throughout the day. Cutting back on classic dehydrating drinks such as coffee and cola is also helpful. So, too, are simple steps, such as having fluids to hand when speaking for long periods, and drinking before, during, and after physical exercise.

sweet breath

Around 85 to 90 per cent of poor-smelling breath is the result of bacteria in the mouth, although chronic sinusitis and nasal problems can also lead to a dreadful odour. Foods that boost the immune system may help to alleviate bacteria and reverse poor breath.

In addition, you can help your mouth to help itself by drinking plenty of water and chewing sugar-free gum made with the bacteria-fighting sweetener, xylitol, when your mouth starts to feel dry. Chewing on parsley, mint, cloves, and fennel seeds can also reduce detrimental bacterial activity.

the tongue

Healthy tongues go largely unnoticed, but one that's under par can look red, swollen, cracked, or discoloured. A lack of certain vitamins, stress, tiredness, a toxin overload, and too little water in the diet can all be reasons for tongue problems. In Chinese medicine, the health of the liver is believed to be reflected in the condition of the tongue. Thus, eating to keep the liver in top condition could have a direct effect on tongue health – which is why a regular supply of good-quality nutrients and keeping a careful eye on alcohol intake are two important steps for maintaining a beautiful mouth.

mouth facts

- Human beings have 32 teeth in a full set.

- A tooth can die when its nerve is damaged. Typically when this happens the pulp becomes infected by bacteria, which means the tooth must be removed.

- Around 750ml (26fl oz) of saliva is produced in the mouth each day.

- Saliva is 97 to 99.5 per cent water and is slightly acidic in composition.

- Saliva contains antibodies and enzymes that naturally help fight tooth decay. It also contains a growth factor, which may help small wounds on the lips to heal when licked.

- Xylitol is a natural sweet substance found in fruits and also in the bark of the birch tree. Research shows that when chewed in sugar-free gum, it reduces bacteria in the mouth and lowers the risk of tooth decay.

- Smoking causes bad breath. If you want to improve your breath, give it up.

- Vague itching, aching, and discomfort can be a sign of periodontal disease, as can loose teeth. If you have any of these symptoms, see your dentist immediately.

mouth
beauty foods

Other decay-fighting foods

Yellow plums and sweets, cheese, milk, water

xylitol chewing gum

promote fresh, cool breath and fight decay

what xylitol chewing gum does

Xylitol-containing chewing gum **protects teeth** from the development of dental decay. This helps to **reduce the need for fillings**. Xylitol in the gum also has a cooling effect in the mouth, freshens the breath and increases saliva flow.

why xylitol chewing gum works

Xylitol is a naturally sweet substance found in the bark of the birch tree. Unlike sugar it does not cause tooth decay. In fact research has shown conclusively that xylitol helps to lower acidity and reduce decay causing bacteria in the mouth, stopping their build up on the teeth. It also encourages remineralization of damaged tooth enamel, and increases saliva production, which washes potential decay forming food debris from around the teeth. Xylitol has also been shown to lower the temperature of the mouth, producing a fresh, cooling effect.

xylitol chewing gum ideas

A range of xylitol containing sugar free gums are available sold both as specialist dental gums and as standard confectionery brands. Chew after meals to reduce acidity and bacterial activity in the mouth.

xylitol watchpoints

Like other Obulk sweeteners such as sorbitol and mannitol found in sugar free chewing gums and sugar free sweets, excess xylitol can cause loose stools when taken in excessive quantities.

what cranberries do

New research suggests that a substance in cranberries may help keep the teeth's **enamel intact**, making it less prone to damage. Cranberries may also **protect the gums** from unsightly plaque accumulation and subsequent bad breath. Cranberries could also play a **gum-strengthening** role, so that the risk of bleeding when eating hard foods or when brushed is reduced.

why cranberries work

Cranberries contain anthocyanins, a type of plant chemical that is able to coat the outside of bacteria, which reduces their ability to stick and cause trouble. Under experimental conditions, these anthocyanidins have been shown to reduce the ability of bacteria to attach themselves to the teeth and gums. This, in turn, may lower the risk of developing plaque, the acid-producing, sticky film of sugar and bacteria that erodes tooth enamel and the gum margins. Anthocyanidins also strengthen blood vessels in the gum.

cranberry serving ideas

The uses of cranberries are limited as a fruit due to their tart flavour. While they can be used whole, chopped, or crushed in sauces, bread, and desserts, cranberry juice is the easiest way of serving. Reduced-sugar and no-added-sugar versions are now available; the latter are mixed with apple juice to improve palatability. Cranberry juice is best served chilled.

cranberry watchpoints

The added sugar and fruit sugars present naturally in mixed cranberry juices mean that their role in dental health should be confined to a sugar-free variety consumed at mealtimes.

cranberries

fight bacteria that causes tooth decay and gum problems

Other gum-strengthening foods

Blueberries, strawberries, raspberries, ginkgo biloba, green tea

parsley

freshens breath and keeps gums pink and strong

what parsley does

The illusion of a beautiful-looking mouth can be spoiled in an instant when the breath is stale. Parsley helps to keep the **breath** smelling **fresh** and sweet. It also supplies nutrients able to **improve** the **strength** and **elasticity** of skin surrounding the lips, helping to retain collagen structure and potentially **preventing fine lines** from forming around the mouth.

how parsley works

Parsley has long been known for its deodorizing properties. This appears to be due to the large amounts of the green pigment chlorophyll, which is thought to combat odours. Parsley is also rich in aromatic essential oils, which help to freshen the breath if chewed after a meal, especially one that has contained garlic. An excellent source of vitamin C, this herb may also protect against mouth lines by deactivating the MMP-1 enzyme that otherwise destroys collagen.

parsley serving ideas

Chew raw following a meal for optimum breath-freshening effects, or include in meals to gain its nutritional benefits. Flat-leafed varieties have a stronger flavour than their curly counterparts. The volatile oils are strong, and so parsley should be added toward the end of cooking or used liberally as a garnish. Use raw in salads, sandwiches, and soups, and as a garnish with fish dishes.

Other virus-fighting foods

Fish, pulses, eggs, red meat, brewer's yeast

chicken

fights the cold-sore virus

what chicken does

Including chicken regularly at mealtimes may play a role in keeping the mouth free from cold sores by helping to maintain the **health** of both the lips and their outer margins. It may also be useful for **reducing** the appearance of **lines** around the mouth. Dark chicken meat particularly can contribute to keeping up good **colour** in the lips, and supplies nutrients needed for the promotion of a fine, smooth texture.

how chicken works

Chicken is rich in a particular protein building-block called lysine, which is known to suppress the growth of the cold-sore-causing herpes simplex virus. Lysine is also instrumental in the formation of collagen which provides the "scaffolding" of skin and may help to lessen the development of fine lines around the mouth. Dark chicken meat supplies iron, which is needed for the formation of the red-blood pigment haemoglobin, which gives lips their seductive red colour.

chicken serving ideas

Chicken can be prepared with everything from red wine or chillies to ginger or teriyaki sauce. Versatile almost to a fault, it can be cooked in a variety of ways, from roasting or grilling to barbecuing or stir-frying; depending on the style of cooking, it can be tasty hot or cold with a selection of hot vegetables or salad ingredients.

chicken watchpoints

To avoid food poisoning, chicken should be stored carefully in the fridge prior to use and cooked quickly once prepared. If serving cold, chicken should be cooled rapidly and then stored immediately in the fridge.

what wheat flakes do

Wheat flakes supply **nutrients** necessary to keep the **tongue in peak condition**, with an **even**, **pinkish** colour and good **texture**. They can also be useful for ensuring that the **lips remain free from swelling** and cracks, especially in the corners of the mouth. Lips chapped through exposure to heat or cold may also benefit by **healing** more swiftly.

why wheat flakes work

Wheat flakes are fortified with riboflavin (vitamin B_2), which is crucial for the health of the mouth. A lack of riboflavin leads to a red, swollen tongue, and also to the breakdown and inflammation of cells in the lips, causing swelling and cracks. In addition, wheat flakes provide zinc and iron needed for rapid and effective healing and for a constant supply of oxygen in the blood to all parts of the mouth.

wheat flake serving ideas

Wheat flakes are best served with chilled milk. Fresh fruits, such as sliced strawberries, whole raspberries, or peach segments, can be added, or the flakes can be topped with yoghurt and grated apple. Wheat flakes can be mixed with oats and dried fruits and nuts to create a muesli, or may be crushed and used in crumble toppings.

wheat flake watchpoints

Wheat flakes should be avoided by anyone with a wheat and gluten intolerance.

wheat flakes

for crack-free lips and a well-conditioned tongue

Other lip-conditioning foods

Fortified bran flakes, chicken, avocado, soya beans, cottage cheese

what co-Q_{10} does

Coenzyme Q_{10}, also known simply as Co-Q_{10}, has been shown to help to keep the **gums** in **peak condition**, bolstering them to **fight infections**, retain their **strength**, **texture**, and **colour**, and to **reduce bleeding** if weaknesses have developed. Regularly taking supplements of Co-Q_{10} can reduce mobility of wobbly teeth and the redness and discomfort associated with gum problems.

why co-Q_{10} works

Co-Q_{10}, a natural substance produced in the body, speeds up the metabolic processes, providing energy to cells, particularly those involved in the repair of wounds. This has a profound effect on the gums, helping to rebuild their structure, heal damaged areas, and stabilize the teeth. Co-Q_{10} also has strong antioxidant properties, working with vitamins C and E to reduce damage by free radicals that enter the mouth through air pollution, cigarette smoke, and passive smoking.

co-Q_{10} serving ideas

Co-Q_{10} is found in some foods, but it needs to be taken in supplement form in order to increase intakes significantly. The recommended level is 50mg twice a day, increasing to 100mg twice daily if treating a gum problem. Co-Q_{10} is also found in mackerel and sardines, both of which can be found in cans or served fresh. Soya beans are another good source, as are peanuts and walnuts.

co-Q_{10} watchpoints

At press time, no side-effects from taking Co-Q_{10} were known.

coenzyme Q_{10}

promotes stable teeth and pink gums

Other gum-protecting foods

Green tea, ginkgo biloba, guavas, strawberries, wheat germ

cheese

lowers acid levels and remineralizes teeth

what cheese does

Cheese in the diet may help to maintain **strong, good-looking teeth** that are able to resist attack from dental decay. It can also play a role in keeping the teeth stable and the **gums pink** and attractive-looking. Eating a small piece of cheese after a meal or snack can have particularly **protective** effects.

Other acid-lowering foods

Milk, water, xylitol-sweetened chewing gum, fromage frais

why cheese works

Cheese is rich in the mineral calcium, needed for the constant renewal and remineralization of the tooth's outer enamel surface. Calcium makes its way to the enamel in the blood supply via the pulpy centre of the tooth. Cheese also contains a protein called casein, which research suggests helps enamel repair itself from the outside following an acid attack in the mouth. Casein seems to attach itself to the tooth's surface, allowing calcium to enter the enamel directly. Cheese also reduces overall mouth acidity.

cheese serving ideas

For direct protective effects, mature, reduced-fat cheese is rich in casein but lower in fat and calories than traditional versions and makes a good option after a meal, when a small chunk can be eaten. To take advantage of its calcium content, serve cheese in sandwiches, in a salad, in sauces, grated on toast, or with fresh fruit.

cheese watchpoints

Cheddar cheese is rich in calcium, but also supplies 412 calories and 34g (1¼oz) of fat per 100g (3½oz) serving. Only small amounts are needed to benefit from its positive effects in the mouth.

Other breath-freshening foods

Fluoridated water, ginkgo biloba, parsley, aniseed, caraway seeds, coriander, fennel seeds

green tea

strengthens enamel, heals gums, and freshens breath

what green tea does

Green tea is believed by Japanese scientists to keep the gums in **peak condition** and to improve them, even in the most severe cases of gum disease. It can also help to **strengthen the enamel** of the teeth and fight against tooth decay. Breath may be **fresher** after drinking green tea, and it may also help to **control the outbreak** of **cold sores** and **mouth ulcers**.

why green tea works

Green tea is packed with potent antioxidant plant nutrients called polyphenols, which, according to research conducted in Japan, promotes the healing of damaged gums. It also appears to reduce the risk of decay through its antibacterial activity and by supplying fluoride. Green tea has direct antiviral effects, helping reduce the activity of the cold-sore virus and working indirectly by enhancing the immune system, making it less prone to attack. Green tea also seems to help heal mouth ulcers.

green tea serving ideas

Green tea is brewed by pouring 225ml (8fl oz) of very hot water over one teaspoon of leaves, leaving for five minutes, then straining and drinking on its own or with meals. Green tea can be chilled, and makes a refreshing beverage served cold. Green tea's polyphenols can be taken in green-tea supplements, which come in capsule and tablet form.

green tea watchpoints

Each cup of green tea contains about 40mg of caffeine, similar to traditional black tea. If trying to cut back on caffeine, limit yourself to one to two cups a day and consider taking supplements instead.

what kava kava does

Plant nutrients called kava lactones are found in the root of the South Pacific kava kava plant, and may help in keeping the **cells in the mouth and lips healthy** by making them better able to **fight infections**. Kava kava may also help to lower the chances of developing ulcers in the mouth and cold sores on the lips.

why kava kava works

The active kava lactones are believed to have an effect on the limbic part of the brain, which regulates emotions. Through exerting a calming influence, kava kava reduces stress and nervousness and improves the chances of a sound night's sleep. In turn, this helps to promote a strong immune system which helps to ward off the bacteria that cause ulcers. A robust immune system also assists the body in fighting the cold-sore virus.

kava kava serving ideas

A traditional drink is made by crushing the kava kava root, adding water or coconut milk, then straining. Dried kava kava can be purchased to make this, but it is more easily available in capsule, liquid, tablet, and tincture form. Herbalists recommend three cups of kava kava tea daily or 250mg of the standardized extract twice to three times daily in supplement form.

kava kava watchpoints

Excessive kava kava may result in a yellowing and dryness of the skin. Kava kava should not be taken by pregnant or breast-feeding women. Excessive doses lead to euphoria and the appearance of drunkenness. Do not take continuously for more than three months. Do not take with alcohol or prescribed medications.

kava kava

reduces stress, boosts natural immunity

Other stress-relieving foods

Chamomile tea, lettuce, bananas, oats, St John's wort, valerian

mouth
beauty diet

Tatty, cracked lips are painful, unsightly, and indicate too little attention to your beauty regime. For a soft, smooth appearance, you need plenty of B vitamins – which can be found in the following three-day beauty diet in fortified breakfast cereals, rye bread, and pasta. The diet also pays attention to the nutrients needed for strong teeth and great gums, such as the calcium that comes from milk and yoghurt, where possible.

To increase your intake of mouth-protecting nutrients, snack on seeds and fromage frais between meals, and sip green tea, which, according to Japanese research, has been shown to deal effectively with even the most problematic gums.

Drinking water regularly throughout the day is crucial to maintain a good saliva flow. Not only will it help wash away debris that is liable to lead to tooth decay, it will also help keep the breath sweet. To make sure your mouth stays healthy, supplement this food plan by keeping parsley or a range of seeds such as aniseed, cardamom, and caraway on hand to chew discreetly at the end of every meal.

3–day mouth diet

	breakfast	lunch	dinner
1	fruity french toast	tuna and spring onion pâté on toasted rye	grilled paprika chicken with sweet-and-sour sauce
2	mango and mint oat whip	quick kedgeree	tomato and parmesan gnocchi
3	cranberry kiss	herby egg scramble	egg noodle stir-fry and teriyaki-style chicken

day 1 *recipes*

fruity french toast

1 egg

pinch of cinnamon

1 tsp brown sugar

1 slice wholemeal bread
sunflower oil

1 tbsp blueberries

2 tbsps low-fat fromage frais

1. Whisk the egg and then add the cinnamon and sugar. Dip the bread into the mixture, coating both sides well. Brush a frying pan lightly with the oil. Add the bread and cook for two to three minutes each side.
2. Mix the blueberries into the fromage frais and use the mixture to top the fried bread while still hot.

grilled paprika chicken with sweet-and-sour sauce

100g (3½oz) skinless chicken breast

salt and freshly ground black pepper

½ tsp paprika

50ml (2fl oz) rice vinegar

1 tbsp castor sugar

100ml (3½fl oz) tomato passata

100g (3½oz) green beans

125g (4½oz) cooked
wholegrain pasta

tuna and spring onion pâté on toasted rye

2 large slices rye bread
sunflower oil

50g (1¾ oz) canned cooked tuna,
drained

2 spring onions, finely sliced

1 tsp Worcestershire sauce

juice of ½ lemon

1 tsp of fresh coriander, chopped

2 tbsps fat-free vinaigrette dressing

freshly ground black pepper

½ garlic clove

1 tsp grain mustard

1 handful prepared salad leaves

2 salad tomatoes, chopped

1. Pre-heat the oven to 200°C/400°F/gas mark 6. Lay the rye bread on a suitable baking sheet and drizzle lightly with the oil. Toast the bread for ten to twelve minutes, or until it becomes crunchy and brittle.
2. In a bowl, add the drained tuna, the spring onions, Worcestershire sauce, lemon juice, chopped coriander, grain mustard, and one tbsp of the fat-free vinaigrette. Mix well using a fork, season with black pepper, and leave to marinate for a few minutes.
3. Rub the toasted rye bread with the garlic clove. Using a fork, spread the tuna mixture on each of the toast slices. Serve with the salad leaves and chopped tomatoes.

1. Season the chicken breast on both sides with a little salt, pepper, and the paprika. Place under a pre-heated grill and cook either side for three to four minutes each.
2. To make the sauce, add the vinegar, sugar, and tomato sauce to a pan and bring to a steady boil. Turn down the heat and leave to simmer for a few minutes.
3. Steam the green beans. Cook the wholemeal pasta according to the packet instructions.
4. When the chicken is cooked through, slice thinly, arrange on the pasta, and pour on the sweet-and-sour sauce. Serve with the green beans on the side.

day 2 *recipes*

mango and mint oat whip

1 small mango

2 tbsps soya yoghurt

a few mint leaves, roughly torn

1 tbsp crunchy muesli

De-seed, peel and chop the mango. Blend with the yoghurt and mint leaves. Put into a bowl and sprinkle with the crunchy muesli. Serve.

quick kedgeree

1 egg

sunflower oil

1 small onion, peeled and chopped

1 tsp curry powder

55g (2oz) cooked kippers, chunked

55g (2oz) cooked brown rice

lemon juice, to taste

parsley, chopped for garnish

2 lemon wedges

1. Hard-boil the egg, then cool, peel, and finely chop. In a pan, add the oil, onion, and curry powder, and sauté gently.
2. When the onion has become opaque, add the kippers, rice, and eggs, then squeeze over some lemon juice. Cook for four minutes.
3. Sprinkle with chopped parsley and serve with lemon wedges.

tomato and parmesan gnocchi

extra-virgin olive oil

1 onion, chopped

1 garlic clove, crushed

1 x 400g (14oz) can tomatoes

a few fresh basil leaves, torn

Worcestershire sauce

4 black and 4 green olives, stoned and quartered

salt and freshly ground black pepper, to taste

1 tsp sugar

300g (10½oz) gnocchi

2 tbsps Parmesan cheese

1. Coat a saucepan lightly with the oil and sauté the onion over a high heat. When soft, add the garlic and sauté for another minute. Stir in the tomatoes, basil, Worcestershire sauce, and olives. Add the salt, pepper, and sugar, and cook for eight minutes.
2. Put the gnocchi into boiling water and cook for four minutes. Drain.
3. Divide between two warmed plates and top with the sauce. Sprinkle with the Parmesan, and serve with a large green salad.

day 3 *recipes*

cranberry kiss

150ml (5fl oz) sugar-free cranberry juice

30ml (1fl oz) orange juice, chilled

fresh lime juice, chilled

Mix together the chilled juices. Before serving, add a squeeze of fresh lime juice. Serve with a breakfast of wholegrain cereal, milk, and fruit.

herby egg scramble

2 mushrooms

1 slice of wholemeal bread

2 large, free-range eggs

2 tbsps milk

salt and freshly ground black pepper

sunflower oil

1 tsp freshly chopped parsley

1 tsp freshly chopped chervil

1. Grill the mushrooms and toast the bread Beat the eggs with the milk, and a tiny pinch of salt and black pepper.
2. Lightly brush a pan with the oil and pour in the egg mixture. Stir over a very low heat until softly scrambled, then throw in the herbs.
3. Serve on the toast accompanied by the mushrooms.

egg noodle stir-fry and teriyaki-style chicken

sesame oil

100g (3½oz) chicken breast, diced

1 tbsp teriyaki sauce

125g (4½oz) dried egg noodles

2 shallots, peeled and finely sliced

1 (each) red, yellow, and green pepper, de-seeded and finely sliced

150g (5½oz) button mushrooms, sliced

½ red chilli, chopped with a pinch of sugar

85g (3oz) fresh bean sprouts

1 tbsp fish sauce

1. Bring a pan of salted water to a boil ready to cook the noodles. Lightly brush a frying pan with the oil and cook the chicken for three to four minutes, then add the teriyaki sauce. Remove from the pan and set aside.
2. Cook the egg noodles according to the packet instructions.
3. Re-heat the frying pan, adding more oil if necessary. Cook the shallots, peppers, mushrooms, and chilli until softened, then add the cooked chicken and bean sprouts, and then the cooked noodles.
4. Mix well, and add the fish sauce. Serve immediately.

mouth
beauty massage

Setting aside time to give special attention to mouth massage exercises could be one of the best anti-ageing routines you invest in. This set of mouth specific massages not only concentrate on smoothing the area directly the around the lips, but firming the muscles of the jaw and chin line which help to give the mouth region definition. Weekly massage around the mouth will help improve circulation and relieve stress to the area helping to reduce the formation of fine lines.

smooth expression lines

1 Tilting your head to the right, stroke with the back of your hands from the collarbone up to the left jaw and ear, one hand following the other.

2 Tilt your head to the left and repeat stroking with the back of your hands up the right side of the neck. The pressure can be firm and you can alter the speed from firm and slow to lighter and faster. Repeat three times.

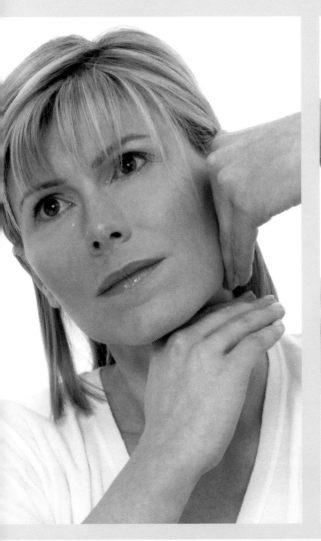

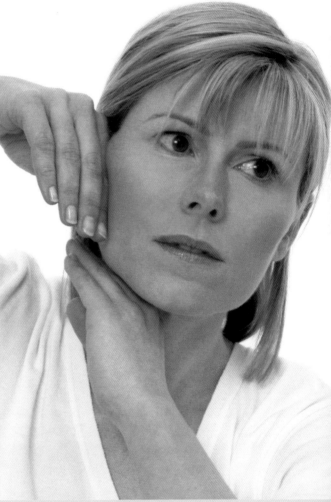

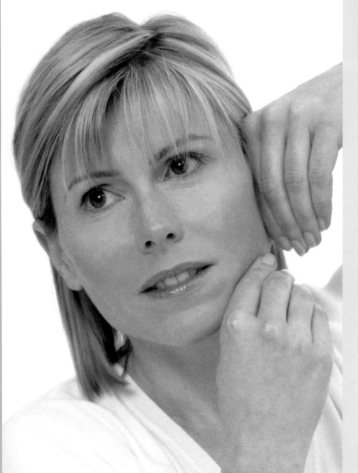

firm the chin

Using your thumbs and the knuckles of your index fingers, pinch along the jaw-line. Start at the centre of your chin and work out toward your ears.

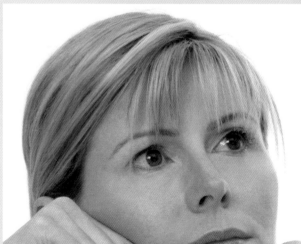

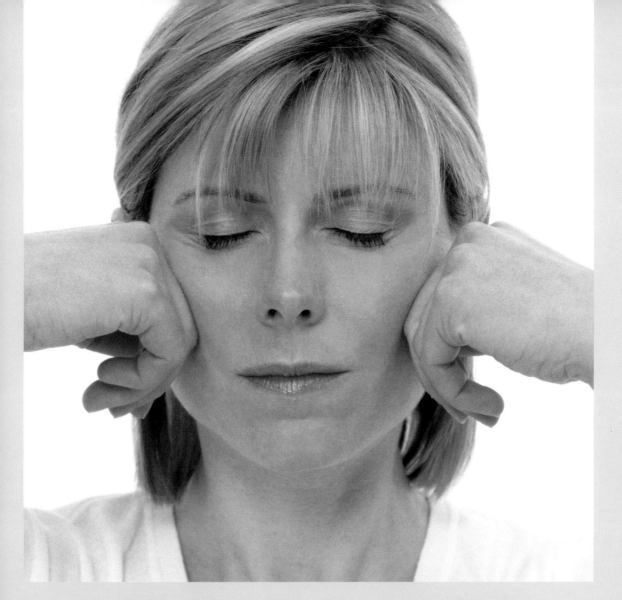

relax the mouth for a bright smile

Form your hands into loose fists and lightly knuckle each cheek. Roll your knuckles upward and outward toward the ears in loose, circular movements, keeping the wrists loose and the hands relaxed. Repeat two to three times.

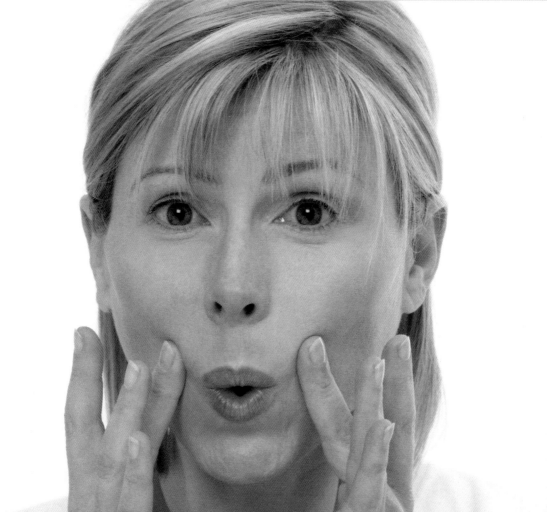

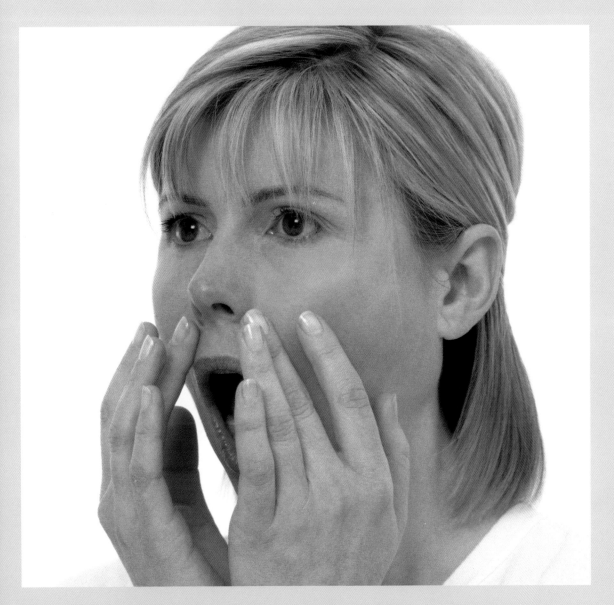

relieve stress around the mouth

Open your mouth wide, as if to say "ah". With the pads of your index fingers, make more circular movements around your open mouth. Start on your chin and work up around the upper lip and then back down again. Repeat.

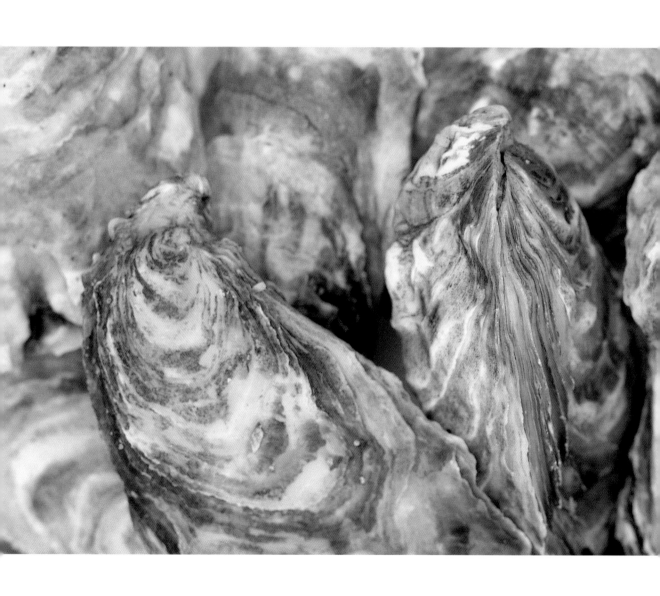

nails

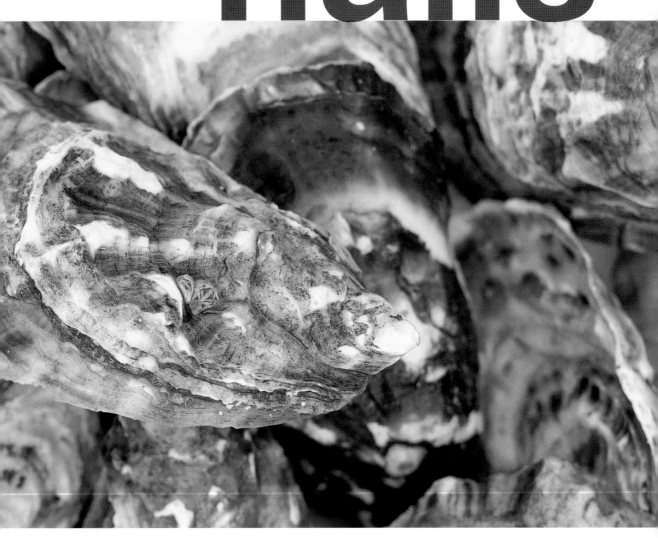

nail care

Nothing gives you a more elegant appearance than well-manicured nails. Designed to help humans make fine movements, nails also protect the ends of fingers and toes from knocks and damage. External care of the hands goes a long way towards enhancing the appearance of nails, but their strength, structure, rate of growth, colour, and texture are all profoundly affected by the things we eat and drink, both on a daily and long-term basis.

nail structure

The part of the nail on show is made up of a tough, dead protein called keratin. This is attached to delicate, underlying skin known as the nail bed, which is richly supplied with blood vessels. A white "half moon" and the area behind it make up the matrix, which is where the nail meets the skin. At the edges of the nail, the skin wraps around and overlaps to form the margin. The cuticle is the thin flap of skin that covers this margin, and it is crucial to nail health, protecting the matrix from water, bacteria, and fungi. Cutting the cuticle into obscurity is not a good idea; first soften it by putting your hands in warm water, and then gently push it back with an orange or cuticle stick.

nail growth

The formation of each new nail begins at the tip of the nail bed, under the skin between the half moon and first finger joint. Here, the cells are soft; as they gradually make their way towards the half moon, they become keratinized, or hardened, with tough, dead keratin cells. By the time they emerge into the outside world as the nail, they are completely dead. In warmer climates, nails grow faster, with those on the fingers growing more rapidly than on the toes. While the nails themselves have no nerves or blood supply, they look pink in colour because of the blood that flows through the vessels in the nail bed underneath.

nail faults

Nails often have small ridges and furrows in them, and trying to buff these out will cause thinning, making them more prone to breaks and splitting. Ridges, furrows, and very defined striations can be due to a lack of certain nutrients, and if this is the case can be reversed by implementing a good diet. Whatever the cause of striations and ridges, a clear nail polish applied before a top coat can help to fill in ridges and give a more even, finished appearance.

nail facts

- Nails grow around 0.5mm per week although this can be reduced to 0.05mm or speed up to 1.2mm, depending on nutrition, temperature, and general health.

- A completely new fingernail can be grown in approximately five to seven months, with those on the middle fingers growing at the fastest rate.

- Nail growth slows with age. Children have the fastest-growing nails and older people the slowest.

- Eating gelatin does not make your nails grow.

- The same nutrients needed for hair growth are needed for nails, and the mineral calcium is particularly important.

- Drinking plenty of water helps keep nails healthy, because nails are around 16 per cent water.

- If you're right-handed, the nails on your right hand will grow fastest. If left-handed, then the opposite is true.

- Nails are dead cells, so they cannot be nourished or fed by rubbing in vitamins and oils. You can, however, help to keep them moisturized by using creams daily.

nail
beauty foods

Other nail-strengthening foods
Fortified breakfast cereals, sardines, eggs, milk

herrings

for better calcium absorption and strong nail structure

what herrings do

Including herrings in the diet, especially during the winter season, can help the body to produce a **strong nail plate**. They may also help ensure a good, **rounded shape** to the nail, an **even thickness**, and a **sturdy structure**. Increasing intakes of oily fish such as herrings, anchovies, mackerel, and pilchards might help to correct spoon-shaped nails.

why herrings work

Herrings are one of the few – and certainly one of the richest – sources of vitamin D in the diet, which is crucial for the absorption of nail-strengthening calcium from the digestive system. We make vitamin D in the skin when exposed to ultraviolet radiation, but stores may not be adequate to last through winter. Herrings and other oily fish are also a good source of iron, a lack of which leads to thin, brittle nails with a concave, spoon shape.

herring serving ideas

Fresh herrings are best grilled or baked. Coating in oatmeal prior to frying is a favourite method in Scotland. Kippers, which are cured herrings, can be grilled and served at breakfast with bread, used to make kedgeree, or made into pâté. Roll-mop herrings are made by sousing fresh herrings in vinegar and are ideal in smorgasbords and salads.

herring watchpoints

Watch out for bones in fresh herrings and kippers, which can cause choking.

garlic

fights infections and promotes growth

Other infection-fighting foods

Spring onions, shallots, leeks

what garlic does

Garlic can work wonders for the nails, helping them grow a **strong nail plate** that stands up to the rigours of daily life; it also helps them look **pink** and **natural**. Garlic helps the body **resist** nail **infections**, which can leave them looking gnarled, thickened, and discoloured.

why garlic works

Garlic can improve the flow of nutrients and oxygen to the nails of both toes and fingers by helping to widen blood vessels. It also keeps nutrients and oxygen needed for optimum nail growth flowing freely, keeping blood vessels free of cholesterol build-ups on their walls. Garlic also contains the phytochemical (*phyto-* means plant) alliin; when garlic is crushed, this turns into allicin, a sulphur-based compound known to thwart bacterial and fungal infections such as athlete's foot.

garlic serving ideas

The benefits of allicin are destroyed during cooking, so garlic is best eaten raw for its preventive and healing properties. Finely chopped, fresh garlic can be added to salad dressings and it is an essential ingredient for hummus. It can also be used in traditional salads such as falafel, and in pesto sauce added to pasta after cooking. Garlic supplements are also available.

garlic watchpoints

Deodorized garlic supplements and enteric-coated versions overcome the problem of "garlic breath" associated with the fresh herb.

Other foods for straight nails

Asparagus, kale, spinach, Brussels sprouts, fortified breakfast cereals

black-eyed peas

promote pink, straight nails

what black-eyed peas do

Black-eyed peas, along with fortified breakfast cereals and beetroot, may contribute to keeping the nails a **soft pink colour**. This pulse, also known as the cow-pea, additionally may help to ensure a good nail **shape** and **texture** by enhancing straight growth without white spots, splits, and breaks.

why black-eyed peas work

Black-eyed peas provide folate, a B vitamin needed for the formation of the red, oxygen-carrying blood pigment haemoglobin, which gives a good colour to the nail bed, and thus the nail that rests on it. Folate and other B vitamins in black-eyed peas help counter stress, which otherwise slows nail growth, makes them brittle, and may lead to white spots.

black-eyed pea serving ideas

After soaking for two to three hours, black-eyed peas should be brought to a boil, then simmered for an hour. They can be used to make bean soups and stews, or served cold in bean salads. Blend with fresh ginger, chilli, garlic, onion, and seasoning to make a tasty bean fritter.

black-eyed pea watchpoints

Soak thoroughly before use, then change the water, bring to the boil and simmer for at least an hour.

what eggs do

Including eggs in the diet is thought to be useful for general **nail-strengthening**, helping nails resist cracks and breaks, making them more **resilient** to everyday changes in temperature, dipping in and out of water, and exposure to detergents. Eggs can also help in the **growth** of young nail cells in the nail matrix.

why eggs work

The yolks of eggs provide the body with the B vitamin biotin. Along with other B-group vitamins, plus vitamins C and E, biotin is used in the formation of the tough nail protein known as keratin. Eggs also supply the body with sulphur-containing amino acids called cysteine and methionine. The sulphurous parts of these proteins are also important ingredients in the development of keratin. In addition, egg yolks supply vitamin D, which is needed for the absorption of calcium.

egg serving ideas

Serve softly boiled for breakfast with bread or toast, or hard-boiled, sliced in sandwiches and salads. Poached eggs can be served on toast, or as a main meal on ham with spinach sauce as eggs Florentine. Scrambled eggs are excellent with smoked salmon, or they can be fried for a traditional hearty breakfast.

egg watchpoints

Avoid cracked eggs and cook before the use-by date. Raw and lightly cooked eggs should not be eaten by children, pregnant women, and anyone who is ill to avoid the risk of salmonella poisoning.

eggs

foster keratin development

Other keratin-building foods

Game, lean beef, cod, scallops, salmon

Other circulation-boosting foods

Garlic, mackerel, tuna, flax seeds, green tea, cinnamon, ginger

ginkgo biloba

promotes good circulation

what ginkgo biloba does

The **speed** with which nails grow may be improved by regularly including ginkgo biloba in the diet. It may also help the development of **stronger nails**, which are less prone to breaks and cracks when knocked and bumped. By increasing circulation, ginkgo also helps ensure that nail cells receive all necessary **nutrients** more efficiently.

how ginkgo biloba works

Standardized extracts from the leaves of the ancient ginkgo biloba tree contain substances known as ginkgolides and bilobides. Studies have shown that these extracts improve the tone and elasticity of blood vessels throughout the body, especially to the extremities, which include the tiny capillaries of the hands and feet. The increase in blood-flow to these areas helps carry protein, energy, vitamins, minerals, oxygen, and water to the developing nail bed.

ginkgo biloba serving ideas

An infusion can be made using 50g (1¾oz) of dried leaves of the ginkgo biloba tree with 500ml (18fl oz) of hot water, to be sipped throughout the day. Ready-made tinctures are also available, along with capsules and tablets containing specific quantities of ginkgolide and bilobide extracts. Up to 240mg of ginkgo biloba extract can be taken daily.

ginkgo biloba watchpoints

Do not use fresh or unprocessed ginkgo biloba leaves to make any infusions or tinctures because they contain strong allergens liable to cause an allergic reaction. Check with your doctor before taking if your are on any form of medication.

oysters

for even, fleck-free nails

what oysters do

Oysters, along with other shellfish, can help in the development of a **smooth**, even nail plate, free from ridges and bumps. They may also help to **clear** new nail growth of **white flecks**. Oysters can play a part in giving the nails a good, defined pink **colour**, helping to differentiate between the main nail and the white tips, and creating a strong, polished look.

why oysters work

One of the richest known sources of zinc, oysters provide a mineral that is vital for the formation of the nail matrix, the part of the nail responsible for continuous, even nail growth. A lack of zinc can cause white flecks to develop. Oysters also provide copper, which, along with iron, is needed to make the bright-red oxygen-carrying blood pigment known as haemoglobin, giving nails a strong pink hue.

oyster serving ideas

Best served fresh with lemon, pepper, and bread and butter, oysters are also delicious when grilled, poached, or fried, with various sauces. Oysters can be added to seafood pasta dishes and paella, seafood soups, and casseroles.

oyster watchpoints

Oysters bought in their shells should be alive. Watch out for half-opened shells and avoid if they are not shiny, fresh smelling, and have a clear liquid free of particles on opening.

what red peppers do

Peppers help keep the nails **hydrated**, and help **avoid brittleness** that inevitably leads to breaks, splits, and peeling. They may also help nails to develop straight from the nail bed. Peppers might also help the body **fight** both bacterial and fungal **infections** to which nails can be prone.

why red peppers work

One large pepper supplies the body with around 250ml (9fl oz) of water, equivalent to a medium-sized glass. Eating raw peppers, celery, melon, and other water-rich foods contributes to overall fluid levels in the body. Nails are composed of sixteen per cent water, and so when levels fall below this amount, they become prone to brittleness, breakage, and peeling. One red pepper also provides huge amounts – nine times the daily requirement – of the immune-boosting vitamin C, which helps fight infections.

red pepper serving ideas

Red peppers taste sweeter than green ones. For maximum beauty-boosting effects, peppers are best served raw in salads, as crudités for dips, as snacks, or in chilled soups such as gazpacho. Cooked swiftly in stir-fries, they lose fewer vitamins and water than if they are roasted. Add them raw to omelettes, or use in casseroles or chilli dishes.

red pepper watchpoints

Avoid peppers with wet stems and blemished skins.

red peppers

fight infections and hydrate nails

Other nail-hydrating foods

Raspberries, strawberries, watermelon, celery, cucumber, lettuce

nail
beauty diet

Ridged, striated, and brittle, thin nails make it hard to achieve a well-polished appearance.
Paying attention to the kinds of foods you eat over the long term can help correct many
common nail problems. Increasing intakes of silicon and calcium is important; both are
found in the following meal plan. Good circulation is also vital, as it is needed to deliver
these and other important nutrients and oxygen to the nail bed. Essential fats found
in oily fish, nuts, and seeds, along with the supplement ginkgo biloba, all enhance blood
flow to the tips of the fingers and toes. This diet also pays attention to providing the
mineral zinc, which helps to clear flecks from the nails, and is found in red meat,
wholegrain cereals, and seeds. It also concentrates on supplying adequate protein
and the B vitamin biotin, both of which are known to be important for the building
of keratin and a strong nail plate. Once again, water is a crucial factor: drink 1.5 to
2 litres (six to nine 8oz glasses) daily to help prevent nails from drying out.

5–day nail diet

	breakfast	lunch	dinner
1	chilli-fried eggs	smoked mackerel and horseradish salad	penne with spicy quorn
2	honey-yoghurt swirl	broccoli and almond soup	grilled chicken with tarragon and garlic
3	poached egg on granary	baked potato with boursin, bacon, and sesame seeds	mustard-pickled herrings
4	sunflower berry bowl	camembert and papaya baguette	grilled duck and roasted pepper pasta
5	fresh blueberry muesli	egg and salad on rye	sweet potato with chilli beef

day 1 *recipes*

chilli-fried eggs

1 slice frozen wholemeal bread

1 tomato

extra-virgin olive oil

2 eggs

1 red chilli, de-seeded and chopped

garlic salt, to taste

parsley, chopped, for garnish

1. Toast the bread from frozen. Cool and toast again to maximize crispness. Cut in half.
2. Slice the tomato in half, drizzle lightly with oil, and grill.
3. In an oil-coated pan, fry the eggs over a medium heat for four minutes. Halfway through frying, add the chilli and garlic salt.
4. When ready, place one egg on top of each half slice of toast, sprinkle with parsley, and serve with the grilled tomato.

penne with spicy quorn

85g (3oz) wholegrain penne

2 spring onions, finely chopped

extra-virgin olive oil

100g (3½oz) Quorn Supreme, cut into strips

½ red chilli

pinch of sugar

100ml (3½fl oz) white wine

100g (3½oz) tomato pasta sauce

sugar, salt, and pepper

juice of ½ lemon

1 small bunch chives, chopped

smoked mackerel and horseradish salad

85g (3oz) peppered smoked mackerel fillet

1 tsp creamed horseradish sauce

1 tsp runny honey

juice of ½ lemon

1 tbsp fat-free vinaigrette dressing

100g (3½oz) cooked new potatoes, sliced

10 cherry tomatoes, halved

1 large bowl prepared salad leaves

salt and freshly ground black pepper

1. Pre-heat the grill. Grill the mackerel skin-side up for two to three minutes. Peel off the skin and scrape off any remaining fatty flesh with a small knife. Set aside.
2. Put the horseradish into a bowl with the honey, lemon juice, and dressing. Whisk well and then add the new potatoes and cherry tomatoes.
3. Add the salad leaves and seasoning and gently mix well.
4. Serve in a suitably sized salad bowl with the warm smoked mackerel flaked over the top.

1. Cook the pasta according to the packet instructions.
2. Sauté the spring onions in a little oil until they begin to soften, then add the Quorn and cook for two or three more minutes. Chop the red chilli with a pinch of sugar to reduce the heat and add to the frying pan. Pour in the white wine.
3. When the wine has reduced, add the tomato sauce and season with a little sugar, salt, and pepper. Drain the pasta, pour into a bowl, then pour on the sauce. Sprinkle with lemon juice and chopped chives to serve.

day 2 *recipes*

honey-yoghurt swirl

100g (3½oz) frozen berries
150g (5½oz) plain yoghurt
1 tbsp runny honey
1 tsp toasted sunflower seeds

Defrost the berries and blend with the yoghurt. Swirl in the honey and top with the sunflower seeds. Serve in a bowl, partnered with a glass of fresh fruit juice.

broccoli and almond soup

extra-virgin olive oil
1 small onion, finely sliced
½ head of broccoli, cut into small florets
1 small potato, peeled and chopped
1 garlic clove, crushed
25g (1oz) flaked almonds
1 small bunch fresh chives, chopped
a few sprigs fresh thyme
600ml (20fl oz) vegetable stock (use an organic stock cube)
salt and freshly ground black pepper
1 slice wholemeal bread

1. Lightly brush a saucepan with oil and sauté the onion. Once opaque, stir in the broccoli and potato. Cook for three to four minutes, then add the garlic and almonds. After one minute add the chives, thyme, and stock.
2. Bring to the boil, then simmer for twelve to fourteen minutes. Blend until smooth, then season to taste and serve with the bread.

grilled chicken with tarragon and garlic

100g (3½oz) skinless chicken breast
salt and freshly ground black pepper
1 tsp sunflower oil
1 tbsp chopped tarragon
200g (7oz) cooked new potatoes
1 tsp grain mustard
100g (3½oz) mange-tout
pinch of sugar
a few fresh mint leaves, chopped

1. Season the chicken with salt and pepper, brush with the oil and place under a pre-heated grill to cook for four to five minutes each side. Halfway through the cooking time, sprinkle with the tarragon.
2. Meanwhile, reheat the cooked new potatoes and then crush them with a fork. Mix in the grain mustard and season with pepper.
3. Cook the mange-tout quickly in either a pan of boiling water or in the microwave. When cooked, add a pinch of sugar and some chopped fresh mint to enhance their taste.
4. Serve the tarragon chicken with the crushed new potatoes and the mint-scented mange-tout on the side.

day 3 *recipes*

poached egg on granary

extra-virgin olive oil
2 mushrooms, sliced
1 tomato, sliced in half
dash of vinegar
1 egg
2 slices granary bread
freshly ground black pepper
parsley, finely chopped for garnish

1. Coat a small frying pan lightly with oil and fry the mushrooms and tomato.
2. Bring a pan of water to the boil; add a dash of vinegar and crack in the egg. Poach for three to four minutes. Meanwhile, toast the bread and cool.
3. Remove the egg from the water and drain. Place on one slice of toast and pile the other high with mushrooms and tomato. Season with black pepper, sprinkle with the parsley, and serve.

baked potato with boursin, bacon, and sesame seeds

1 baking potato, washed
juice of 1 lemon
freshly ground black pepper
2 tsps Boursin Light
1 extra-lean rasher bacon
1 tsp toasted sesame seeds

1. Bake the potato and scoop it out of its skin, reserving the latter. Drizzle the soft potato with the lemon juice and mix in with a fork; do the same with plenty of black pepper and the boursin.
2. Grill the bacon until crispy, then break into small pieces. Pile the potato mix back into the skin. Sprinkle with the bacon pieces and sesame seeds. Serve with a large mixed salad.

mustard-pickled herrings

extra-virgin olive oil
100g (3½oz) raw carrots, peeled and grated
250g (9oz) beetroot, peeled and grated
salt and freshly ground black pepper
lemon juice, to taste
200g (7oz) mustard-pickled herrings
2 slices dark rye bread

1. Sauté the carrot in a little of the oil for two to three minutes, then stir in the beetroot and cook until both are soft. Season with salt, black pepper and a squeeze of lemon juice.
2. Roll up the herrings and serve with the beetroot and carrot mixture and bread.

day 4 *recipes*

sunflower berry bowl

100g (3½oz) mixed frozen berries
100g (3½oz) plain fromage frais
1 tbsp wheat germ
1 tbsp honey-roast sunflower seeds

Defrost the berries and stir into the fromage frais along with the wheat germ. Sprinkle with the sunflower seeds and serve.

camembert and papaya baguette

1 small French baguette
55g (2oz) Camembert
½ papaya, peeled and sliced
freshly ground black pepper
watercress

1. Split the baguette and spread with the Camembert. Add the sliced papaya and season with pepper.
2. Top with watercress and serve with fresh fruit juice.

grilled duck and roasted pepper pasta

1 red pepper, halved and de-seeded
½ yellow and ½ orange pepper, de-seeded
1cm (½ inch) ginger root, peeled and grated
½ bunch of spring onions, finely sliced
2 tbsps soy sauce
2 tbsps lemon juice
2 tsps white wine vinegar
1 tbsp clear honey
2 duck breasts
200g (7oz) dried wholegrain spaghetti

1. Grill the peppers until their skins are charred, then put them in a plastic bag and leave for ten minutes.
2. Whisk together the ginger, spring onions, soy sauce, lemon juice, vinegar, and honey. Grill the duck breasts for ten minutes each side and cook the pasta.
3. Peel the peppers and cut them into strips. Remove the skin and fat from the duck breasts and slice. Mix the duck with the peppers and dressing; stir well. Drain the pasta and serve with the duck and pepper sauce.

day 5 *recipes*

fresh blueberry muesli

100g (3½oz) fresh blueberries
25g (1oz) fruit-and-nut muesli
chilled milk

Mix the blueberries with the muesli in a large bowl and pour on plenty of chilled milk.

egg and salad on rye

2 slices rye bread
mayonnaise, to taste
mustard, to taste
watercress
1 tomato, sliced
1 hard boiled egg, peeled and sliced
freshly ground black pepper

1. Spread the rye bread with mayonnaise, then add the mustard, watercress, and slices of tomato.
2. Place the slices of egg on top, season with black pepper, and top with the other piece of rye bread. Serve with a long, cool, spicy tomato juice.

sweet potato with chilli beef

1 large pink sweet potato, washed
salt and freshly ground black pepper
½ medium onion, finely chopped
½ red chilli, finely chopped
extra-virgin olive oil
70g (2½oz) lean minced beef
1 tsp tomato purée
200ml (7fl oz) tomato pasta sauce
1 tbsp chopped parsley
1 ripe plum tomato, sliced
1 tbsp virtually fat-free fromage frais

1. Prick the sweet potato with a fork, then rub salt into the skin for a crispy finish. Microwave for around seven to eight minutes or in the oven for around twenty-five to thirty minutes.
2. Sauté the onion and chilli in a little oil for one minute. Season the minced beef and add to the pan; cook gently for another minute. Add the tomato purée, sauce, and parsley. Simmer gently for five to six minutes.
3. Slit the top of the cooked sweet potato and squeeze gently to open. Spoon in the chilli beef, and serve with a spoonful of fromage frais, the sliced plum tomato, and a mixed salad.

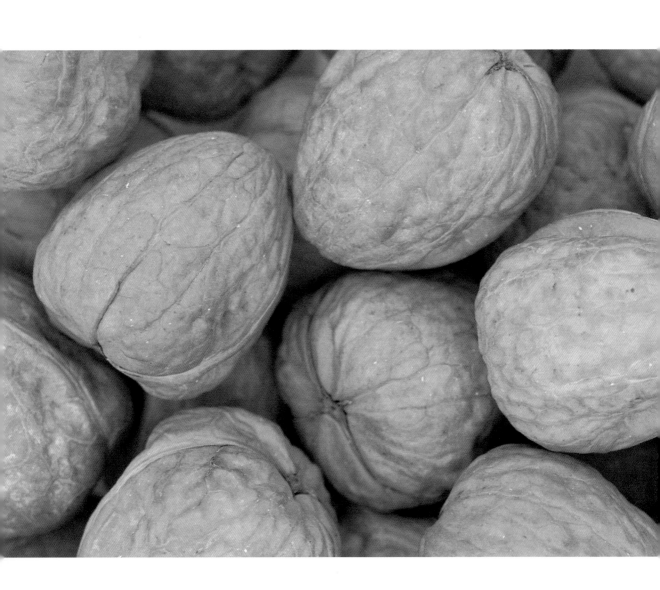

hair

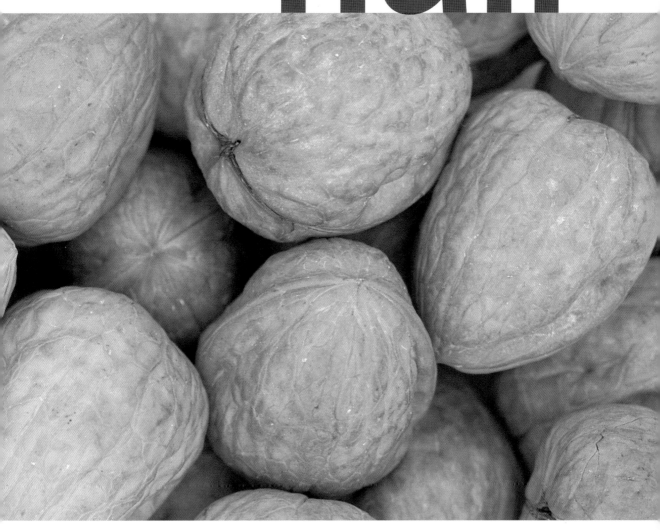

hair care

Hair helps protect the head from sunlight and keeps in body heat. If it is in great shape, hair can also make us feel like a million dollars. To keep it in condition, however, shampoos, conditioners, and hair-care products must be combined with a nutrient-packed eating plan.

how hair grows

Each hair grows from a follicle that sits snugly in the nutrient-rich part of the skin.

At the bottom of the follicle lies the root. As the follicle makes new hair cells, old ones are pushed upward; as they reach the surface of the skin, like nail cells, they become "keratinized", or hardened, and die. So while the hair we see is essentially dead, its roots and follicles are very much alive. Although it is possible to improve the texture and condition of hair through products and treatments applied externally, the key to growing plenty of good-quality hair lies in ensuring that the root and follicle are in good condition. This can be achieved only from within, and is affected by hormone levels, blood supply, and overall health, all of which, in turn, are affected by the foods and drinks we consume.

Hair tends to grow at around 1.75cm (¾ inch) a month, with each hair follicle going through a cycle of growth lasting from three to five years. This growth phase is followed by a short transitional phase, then by a resting phase, during which the hair falls out. At any one time, around fifteen per cent of the hair follicles are in their resting phase, while the others are actively growing. The active period of growth depends a lot on each individual's genetic make-up. Under ideal conditions, hair grows at its fastest from the teen years to the forties, after which point things begin gradually to slow down. It is usual to shed about eighty hairs from our heads a day, replacing them in equal numbers, although this process decreases with age so that hair appears thinner. Thinning also occurs when the diet is short on nutrients and your life is long on stress.

losing your hair

If lots of hair follicles rest at the same time, inevitably they also shed at the same time, leading to quite significant losses. This kind of disruption to growth and rest cycles can be a sign that something is at odds in the body. It could, for example, be triggered by imbalanced hormone levels, something that can be caused by stress. Stress factors can be improved through taking stock of your lifestyle and by bolstering intakes of certain B vitamins. An underactive thyroid gland and its subsequent reduction in the production of the hormone thyroxine can also be responsible for increased hair loss, a problem that iodine-rich foods may help. A lack of certain nutrients in the foods we eat can also trigger hair loss. A gradual or sudden drop in intakes of iron, for instance, is known to be a cause of thinning hair. Anyone deciding to remove meat, a good source of easily absorbed iron, from the diet should be especially aware of ways to replace this vital nutrient from vegetable sources to ensure that hair remains in peak condition.

While improving vitamins and minerals in the diet can help to nourish regular growth and rest cycles of hair follicles, it is also vital to eat adequate amounts of protein-rich foods such as fish, chicken, dairy products, pulses, nuts, and meat alternatives, such as Quorn®. Having some protein at every meal will help ensure adequate intakes. Keeping the gut in good condition is vital, too. If the digestive system is having trouble absorbing nutrients, then however great your intake, the goodness simply will not be absorbed into the blood or be delivered to nourish hair follicles. Regularly including probiotic drinks and yoghurts containing "good" bacteria can help keep and restore the gut to full absorptive health, especially following a course of antibiotics.

Sustained loss of more than one hundred hairs a day may indicate a more serious health problem. It could be attributed to taking too much vitamin A in supplement form (more than 30,000mg over a long period), or to a condition known as alopecia areata, which leads to localized bald patches. While this problem can clear up without treatment within six to twelve months, if heavy hair loss persists, see your doctor or health-care professional.

dieting disasters

Cutting back on calories almost inevitably means compromising on nutrients, and regular "yo-yo" dieting can seriously affect hair health. The effects are most pronounced when attempts to lose weight turn into eating disorders, in which significant weight reduction is accompanied by excessive hair loss and thinning. Avoiding crash-dieting is vital for the maintenance of healthy hair follicles, and it is never too late to begin nourishing them back into shape. A steady stream of nutrients on a daily basis can get them firing on all cylinders within two to three months, and within a year can lead to significant improvements in the health and look of hair.

colour

Natural hair colour is determined by melanin, the same pigment that gives skin its varying shades. Melanin sits in the hair root and is transferred to the central part of the hair shaft as it grows. Various proportions of melanin pigments, which are yellow, brown, black, and rust-coloured, combine to give hair a wide range of colours, from sunkissed blonde to kohl black or vibrant red. Grey hair is white hair interspersed with normal-coloured hair.

White hair results from a reduction of melanin production in the root. Since melanin gives hair not only its colour but also helps it to retain moisture, "greying" leads to loss of hair texture, often causing it to become finer. That it seems wirier is because oil glands also reduce their activity, making the hair drier still. A reduction in melanin production may be due to a poor intake of the mineral copper, and increasing intakes in this instance may help to restore and maintain a good natural colour.

scalp

Once the shaft of a hair has been pushed out of the skin, maximizing its appearance is down to regular care and keeping the scalp in good condition. Skin cells on the scalp are constantly shed. If hair is not washed regularly, loose cells can become glued in place by oil and crumble off as dandruff. If dandruff persists, it can be due to a skin condition such as eczema or psoriasis, both of which may improve by increasing intakes of essential fatty acids found in oily fish, nuts, and seeds. A lack of vitamin A may also be a cause.

hair facts

- Your genes determine the number of hair roots you have, and these neither increase nor decrease throughout life.

- Hair tends to grow faster in warmer climates.

- Millions of hairs are scattered over the body. There are around 10,000 of them in the scalp.

- The way in which hair grows from its root determines whether it is straight, wavy, or curly.

- Different sizes and shapes of the hair roots are what lead to fine or thick hair.

- Melanin pigments help protect the hair from ultraviolet damage from the sun's rays, just as they do in skin.

- Melanin pigments in hair are called eumelanin, which leads to brown and black shades of hair; phaemomelanin, which leads to yellow and red shades; and oxymelanin, which leads to very blonde hair.

- Sustained loss of more than 100 hairs a day may indicate a problem.

hair
beauty foods

Other root-nourishing foods

Mackerel, dark chicken and turkey meat, red meat, fortified breakfast cereals, dark-green vegetables, sesame seeds

sardines

nourish the root to promote regular growth

what sardines do

Including sardines in the diet may help **reduce** both the **loss** of hair and the appearance of **thinning** by encouraging regular growth of each hair follicle. Sardines and other oily fish can also assist in maintaining the **health** of the **scalp**, keeping it well-hydrated, flexible, and resistant to dryness and flaking.

why sardines work

Sardines supply the body with easy-to-absorb haem iron, a lack of which reduces oxygen and nutrient supplies to the hair root, resulting in interrupted growth cycles of each follicle. The rich omega-3 fatty acids this fish contains help to promote the health of skin on the scalp, protecting it from water loss and dryness. Sardines are also an excellent source of protein, which is needed for the production of the hair's tough outer keratin coating.

sardine serving ideas

Sardines are best fresh and cooked whole, either baked, grilled, pan-fried, or barbecued. Serve with rough, crusty, fresh bread, a tomato and basil salad, and add a squeeze of lemon juice and some freshly ground black pepper for a simple supper. Canned sardines come in oil and tomato sauce and can be mixed with balsamic vinegar and used in salads, on toast, and in sandwiches.

sardine watchpoints

Buy as fresh as possible and avoid fish with dull, flat eyes, flabby flesh, or an odd smell. If canned, make sure cans are undamaged.

what crab does

Crab can be involved in maintaining the general **strength** and **resilience** of individual hair structure, giving it good **flexibility** to avoid breaking easily when washing, drying, and brushing. Crab may also have an important part to play in helping hair strands retain their natural **pigmentation** as we age, possibly helping to slow the rate at which hair turns grey.

why crab works

Crab provides the body with copper. While a lack of this mineral in a balanced diet is unusual, if intakes are low, the hair becomes very brittle, with individual strands starting to grow in a corkscrew and taking on a twisted appearance. Eyebrows are also affected, and become tangled and unkempt. Copper is also needed for the manufacture of melanin. Crab boosts intakes of the protein building-blocks methionine and cysteine, which are needed for the development of the keratin that forms the tough outer coating of the hair.

crab serving ideas

Fresh crab is the most nutritious, and can be bought ready-dressed in its shell; serve cold with salad or in sandwiches. Crab meat can also be added to pilaf, served au gratin, or baked with vegetables such as avocado. Crab can be made into a bisque, and makes a tasty addition to seafood soup.

crab watchpoints

When buying cooked whole crab, the limbs should be intact and not discoloured, and when lifted there should be no sound of water. Use immediately, as crab meat spoils rapidly.

crab

retains hair pigment and boosts strength

Other colour-nourishing foods

Oysters, sunflower seeds, cashew nuts, almonds

Other growth-promoting foods

Seaweed, red and grey mullet, whiting, cod, mussels

haddock

promotes strong hair and regular growth cycles

what haddock does

Haddock can play a role in the creation of a strong head of hair. Although the thickness of individual hairs is determined by genetics, this fish may help to **reduce** problems with general **thinning**. Haddock may also be of help in ensuring that each hair shaft is as **robust** as possible, reducing the chances of fragility and the risk of snapping.

why haddock works

This nutritious white fish supplies the body with iodine, a trace mineral essential for the maintenance of the thyroid gland. A lack of iodine leads to an underactive thyroid, which in turn reduces the activity of hair follicles and slows the rate of hair growth. It also leads to the development of weakened individual strands. Haddock provides a good range of B vitamins needed to combat stress and stress-related hair loss, plus protein that is crucial for a strong keratin coating of each strand.

haddock serving ideas

The fine texture and delicate, slightly sweet flavour of haddock means that it can be baked, grilled, or fried as whole fillets. Cooked and flaked, it is great in fish pies and curries, and can be used to make fishcakes served with various sauces and lightly steamed vegetables in season.

haddock watchpoints

Never buy haddock that smells unpleasant, or has eyes that are not bright and moist, and skin that isn't firm and moist.

Other growth-promoting foods
Oysters, wholemeal bread, red meat, sesame seeds, horsetail

oatcakes

nourish the roots for optimal strength

what oatcakes do

Optimum growth rates may be more achievable when including oatcakes and oat-based foods in the diet. They may improve the **strength** of individual strands. A **thick appearance** may also be more achievable, and the risk of thinning and hair loss reduced. Oatcakes help to **nourish** and keep the scalp in good condition and free from flakiness.

why oatcakes work

Oatcakes provide zinc, a lack of which causes the hair to become excessively fragile and sparse on the scalp. They also supply iron, which is necessary for oxygen to be transported to the hair roots. Oatcakes are one of the few sources of the trace mineral silicon, thought to be important for normal hair structure, along with a range of B vitamins needed for good scalp condition, and for soothing frayed nerves which might otherwise contribute to stress-related hair loss.

oatcake serving ideas

Oatcakes can be used as a substitute for bread and crispbreads. They make an excellent base for everything from marmalade or jam at breakfast to savoury spreads with cheese and pâté. Oatcakes travel well and make good accompaniments to soups and salads, and they can be eaten alone as a nutritious, carbohydrate-rich snack.

oatcake watchpoints

Some oatcakes are higher in fat than others. If this is the case, avoid adding margarine or butter.

what walnuts do

Walnuts may help the hair to retain its **natural colour**, **moisture** levels, and **texture** as we age. Some herbalists claim that they actually reverse the greying process. Walnuts can help keep the dermal layer of the skin of the scalp well-supplied with both oxygen and nutrients to feed the roots, keep the follicle in good shape, and encourage regular growth of strong, textured hair.

why walnuts work

Walnuts provide the body with copper needed for the production of the melanin pigments that gives hair its colour and helps it remain hydrated and thick. They also contain iron, a lack of which may be one cause of hair loss and thinning. Research indicates that walnuts help reduce the build-up of cholesterol on blood-vessel walls, which promotes good blood flow, including that to the head and scalp. Omega-6 fatty acids, needed for a healthy scalp, are also present in walnuts.

walnut serving ideas

Ripe walnuts are great eaten straight from the shell as a snack. They go particularly well with cheese, apples, and savoury biscuits. When ground, they make an excellent addition to traditional pesto sauce for pasta, and in France they are used in soups and sauces. Walnuts may be put into ice-cream and baklava, and when broken, they add a distinctive flavour to muesli mixes.

walnut watchpoints

Anyone with nut allergies should avoid walnuts. Those watching their weight should take into account this nut's high calorie and fat content, and limit intakes to a handful a day.

walnuts

help retain hair pigmentation

Other pigment-protecting foods

Mussels, crab, whiting, liver, pulses

what pumpkin seeds do

Regularly eating pumpkin seeds may help to keep the scalp **well-moisturized** and free from excessive oil, dryness, or flaking. They can also play a part in helping the hair **grow** at its maximum speed, as well as supplying the **nutrients** necessary for each hair to develop a strong keratin coating, which reduces the chances of it becoming brittle and breaking easily.

why pumpkin seeds work

Pumpkin seeds are bursting with an array of hair- and scalp-nourishing nutrients. While their good iron levels keep up oxygen supplies to the roots and help prevent hair loss, the protein they supply helps build the hair's protective keratin coating. Pumpkin seeds are also rich in zinc, which helps guard against fragility, while their omega-3 and omega-6 fatty acids are crucial for the health of the sweat and hair follicles, and in keeping the scalp watertight to reduce dry patches.

pumpkin seed serving ideas

Found inside mature pumpkins, the seeds need to be dried either in direct sunlight or in the oven. When the shell is removed, pumpkin seeds can be used fresh or roasted in a little oil and added to salads or muesli mixes, and sprinkled over fruit salads. Pumpkin seeds can be added to bread and fruit-cake mixes, and scattered over soups and casseroles.

pumpkin seed watchpoints

Store seeds in a clear-glass, airtight jar in the fridge to retain freshness for up to six months.

pumpkin seeds

promote a healthy, nourished scalp

Other scalp-conditioning foods

Mackerel, sardines, tuna, flax seeds, chia seeds

guavas

foster follicle health and scalp protection

what guavas do

Uninterrupted, optimum **growth** of individual hair strands from their follicles can be assisted by a diet rich in fruits such as guavas. They may also help ensure the skin of the **scalp** is in **good condition**, that hair grows in a normal pattern, and that it develops its own built-in **protection** from burning when exposed to short bursts of sunlight.

how guavas work

Guavas are among the richest providers of vitamin C, which is needed to keep capillary walls flexible and a regular supply of nutrients flowing to the hair root. Adequate vitamin C is also vital for the health of the skin; a lack causes hair follicles to become blocked with keratin, a process that forces hairs to grow in a corkscrew shape. Guavas' pink colour comes from carotene, which may help protect the skin of the scalp from burning when exposed to the sun's ultraviolet radiation.

guava serving ideas

The pink-fleshed guava is excellent eaten raw, when the fruit is cut lengthways, sprinkled with fresh lime juice, and simply scooped with a teaspoon from the skin. The fruit can also be peeled and served on a platter with cheeses, or sliced and added to fruit salad. Puréed guavas can be made into ice-cream, sorbets, and smoothie drinks.

guava watchpoints

Fresh is always preferable to canned, because the latter has been heat-treated, reducing the vitamin C levels to virtually zero. The carotene will, however, have remained intact.

Other follicle-nourishing foods

Berries, oranges, peppers, papayas, carrots, sweet potatoes

hair
beauty diet

Brittle, thinning hair lacks lustre, body, and condition. To remedy basic problems, return flexibility, and encourage regular and integrated growth of individual hair strands, the roots and follicles need constant feeding with the right nutrients. The following diet is bursting with copper-rich foods such as crab to help retain your hair's natural colour, moisture levels, and texture. It also contains oily fish such as sardines, which supply iron needed to prevent hair loss and thinning associated with anaemia. For each hair strand to grow in a regular cycle at its maximum rate, good intakes of iodine are essential. To this end, foods such as haddock are on the menu.

Stress plays havoc with all aspects of hair health, so well-known stress relievers such as oats are recommended for breakfast. You can give yourself a helping hand to lower stress by adding St John's wort supplements or valerian tea to your health programme. As with any beauty regime, it is vital to drink plenty of water. Aim for between 1.5 to 2 litres (between six to nine 8oz glasses) of water a day.

day 2 *recipes*

toasted sesame and apricot porridge

40g (1½oz) porridge oats
140ml (4½fl oz) milk
40g (1½oz) ready-to-eat apricots
runny honey
1 tsp toasted sesame seeds

1. Mix the porridge with the milk and apricots. Microwave for 90 seconds on full power, or cook on the stove according to the packet instructions.
2. Allow to stand for one minute. Serve drizzled with honey and sprinkled with the sesame seeds.

caesar light

1 large slice wholemeal bread
extra-virgin olive oil
1 hard-boiled egg, chopped
½ garlic clove, crushed
1 tbsp reduced-fat caesar dressing
2 tsp lemon juice
salt and freshly ground black pepper
70g (2½oz) cooked skinless chicken breast, cut into strips
1 garlic clove, cut in half
1 head cos lettuce, washed and cut into chunks
1 tbsp freshly grated Parmesan cheese

1. Pre-heat the grill to maximum. Drizzle the bread with a little oil and grill until toasted thoroughly on each side.
2. In a bowl, mix together the egg, crushed garlic, caesar dressing, lemon juice, salt, and pepper. Whisk well. Add the chicken.
3. Rub the toast with the freshly cut garlic clove, dice into small croûtons, and add half to the chicken. Mix in the lettuce, then serve in a bowl and top with the remaining croûtons.
4. Sprinkle with the Parmesan and black pepper. Serve with a glass of fresh fruit juice.

grilled sardines with balsamic tomato salad

4 large sardines, cleaned
extra-virgin olive oil
juice of 2 lemons
freshly ground black pepper
4 tomatoes, cut into wedges
1 handful fresh basil leaves, torn
balsamic vinegar
crusty bread

1. Run the sardines under water, then drizzle with a little oil. Sprinkle with lemon juice to taste and season with black pepper. Place under a hot grill for three to four minutes each side.
2. Arrange on a warm serving dish. Mix the tomato wedges with the torn basil leaves. Sprinkle with balsamic vinegar and season with black pepper. Serve with the sardines and bread, using more lemon juice on the sardines just before eating, if desired.

day 3 *recipes*

peaches with wheat flakes

40g (½oz) wheatflakes

1 ripe peach, cut into slices

chilled milk

1 tbsp pumpkin seeds

1. Put the wheat flakes in a bowl and add the peach slices.
2. Pour on the milk, sprinkle with the pumpkin seeds, and serve.

mexican bean dip with toasted pitta wedges

1 tbsp chopped shallots

100g (3½oz) tinned kidney beans, drained

1 garlic clove, crushed

1 tbsp fat-free set Greek yoghurt

½ tsp paprika

a few sprigs fresh coriander

juice of ½ lemon

a few drops Tabasco sauce

salt and freshly ground black pepper

1 wholemeal mini pitta

2 carrots

1 stick of celery

½ cucumber

a few leaves baby gem or cos lettuce, to serve

1. Put the chopped shallots, kidney beans, and garlic into either a food processor or small kitchen blender. Add the set yoghurt, paprika, coriander, lemon juice, and Tabasco sauce. Blend until smooth and season to taste with a little salt and lots of pepper. Add more Tabasco if you want a spicier kick to the dip.
2. Meanwhile, toast the wholemeal pitta and cut into wedges to serve next to the Mexican dip.
3. Peel and cut the vegetables into chunky strips, and place in iced water to give them a slight crunch.
4. Remove vegetables from the water before serving, place on some salad leaves with the toasted pitta wedges, and serve with the dip.

spanish-style marinated salmon

50g (2oz) very fresh salmon, cut into thin slices

salt and freshly ground black pepper

zest and juice of 1 lime

1 shallot, peeled and finely chopped

4 small cornichons or 1 gherkin, finely chopped

1 tsp capers, finely chopped

1 tbsp fat-free salad dressing

a few fresh basil leaves, chopped

1 wholemeal mini-pitta

1 small cos lettuce, washed and torn into strips

1 green pepper, finely sliced

1 yellow pepper, finely sliced

2 ripe plum tomatoes, thinly sliced

1. Season the salmon, brush with the lime zest and juice, then leave to marinate in the fridge.
2. Mix the shallot, cornichons, and capers together. Place in a small bowl and add the dressing and basil.
3. Remove the fish from the fridge. Pour any extra lime juice into the caper dressing.
4. Combine the lettuce, peppers, and tomato, then add the dressing. Mix the salmon with the salad and serve with the warmed pitta.

day 4 *recipes*

guava shake

1 guava

150ml (5fl oz) milk

50g (2oz) probiotic yoghurt

crushed ice

1 mint leaf, for garnish

1. Cut the guava in half and scoop out the soft insides.
2. Blend with the milk and yoghurt until smooth. Pour into a chilled glass containing crushed ice. Serve garnished with a mint leaf.

crab and lemon salad sandwich

100g (3½oz) fresh or canned cooked white crab meat

salt and freshly ground black pepper

juice of ½ lemon

drop of Tabasco sauce

2 slices wholemeal bread

a few fresh leaves coriander

50g (2oz) cooked sweetcorn kernels

½ red and ½ green pepper, de-seeded and finely chopped

1 spring onion, finely chopped

a small piece cucumber, finely chopped

1. Pick through the crab meat to make sure that there are no shell fragments left. Season with plenty of freshly milled black pepper, lemon juice, Tabasco, and, if fresh crab, a tiny pinch of salt.
2. Toast the wholemeal bread and cool. It must be crispy to avoid the crab meat making it soggy.
3. Snip the coriander leaves into a glass, then mix with the crab meat and sweetcorn.
4. Combine the peppers, spring onion, and cucumber pieces. Spread the fresh crab mixture onto the toast, top with the pepper salad, and serve straight away.

tikka lamb kebabs

50g (2oz) fat-free set Greek yoghurt

pinch of ground cumin

pinch of turmeric

pinch of garam masala

1 tsp chopped fresh coriander

salt and freshly ground black pepper

1 tbsp fresh lemon juice

1 tsp grated fresh ginger

1 garlic clove, crushed

4 button mushrooms

200g (7oz) cooked new potatoes

70g (2½oz) extra-lean lamb escalope, cut into cubes

1. Pre-heat the grill to maximum. In a bowl, mix together the yoghurt, spices, fresh coriander, salt, pepper, lemon juice, ginger, and garlic until a smooth paste is formed.
2. Pour the paste over the mushrooms, potatoes, and lamb. Once coated, thread the lamb, potato, and mushroom pieces onto kebab skewers. If using bamboo skewers, soak them in water prior to using, so that they don't burn.
3. Grill for eight to 10 minutes, turning over once. Serve with mixed salad leaves.

day 5 *recipes*

walnut bread with honey

2 slices walnut bread
honey
1 handful raisins

1. Spread the bread with honey and add the raisins.
2. Serve with a glass of freshly squeezed orange juice.

roasted bulgar wheat salad with crab

4 level tbsp bulgar wheat

pinch of ground cumin, ground coriander, and turmeric

½ red pepper, ½ yellow pepper and ½ green pepper, de-seeded and finely diced

85g (3oz) cooked sweetcorn

1 handful baby spinach leaves, shredded

300ml (10fl oz) vegetable stock (use an organic stock cube)

juice of ½ lemon

100g (3½oz) cooked prawns

carrot and ginger soup with tofu

extra-virgin olive oil
1 medium onion, peeled and chopped
3 medium carrots, peeled and finely chopped
½ garlic clove, crushed
1 tsp grated fresh ginger
salt and freshly ground black pepper
85g (3oz) plain tofu
600ml (20fl oz) vegetable stock (use an organic stock cube)
1 tbsp virtually fat-free plain fromage frais
2 large slices rye bread

1. Coat a medium-sized saucepan lightly with oil and place on a moderate heat.
2. Add the onions, carrots, garlic, and fresh ginger, and cook for two to three minutes.
3. Once the vegetables have softened slightly, add a little salt, lots of pepper, and the tofu pieces. Stir well and add the vegetable stock. Bring to the boil, then turn down the heat to a gentle simmer.
4. Simmer for twelve to fifteen minutes, then blend in a liquidizer or food processor until smooth. Adjust the seasoning, if necessary. Add a good tbsp of fromage frais or set Greek yoghurt to each bowl.
5. Warm the rye bread – and serve.

1. In a non-stick frying pan, heat the wheat and spices until the wheat starts to turn golden and produces a nutty smell – about five to six minutes.
2. Meanwhile, combine the peppers and sweetcorn and add to the spinach. Once the wheat has started to roast, add the vegetable stock. Cover, and turn down the heat; in four to five minutes, the wheat should have absorbed all the stock.
3. Add the wheat to the spinach and pepper mixture, mix well, then add the fresh lemon juice and cooked prawns, and season to taste.
4. Serve with mixed salad leaves.

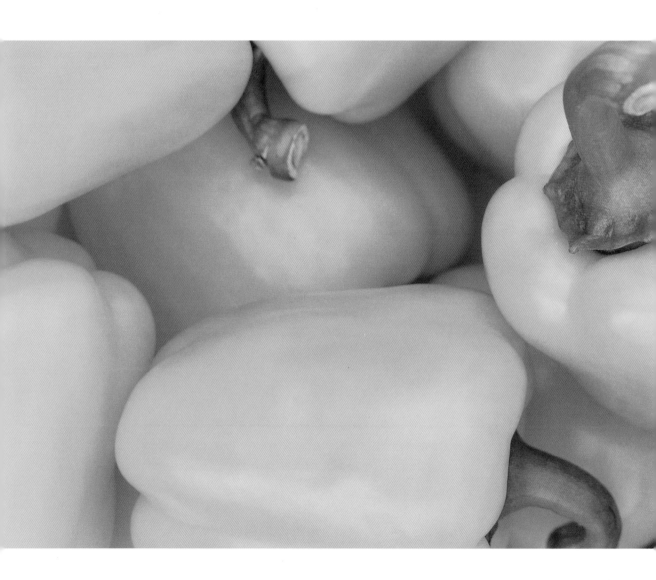

eyes

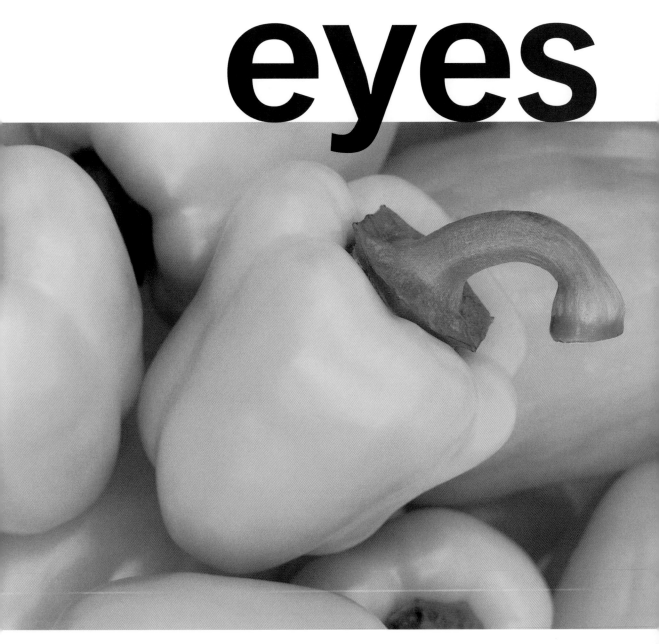

eye care

There is no doubt that great eyes are a huge asset on the beauty front. Throughout the centuries, women the world over have known the importance of a seductive flutter. To sparkle, glisten, and draw attention to your face, the lids, lashes, brows, and tear glands all need to be in great shape. While "this season's colours" and the latest thickening mascara can certainly enhance the eyes, no amount of make-up can camouflage a tired and lacklustre appearance lurking beneath it.

In the West, eyes may be known as the "windows to the soul", but in Chinese medicine, a skilled physician can determine much about our overall physical health through a thorough eye examination. Understanding a little of the structure of the eye makes it easier to see how the foods and drinks you choose can affect not just the way your eyes appear, but also help to put the brightness back and keep them in great condition for years to come.

the eyes

Only around one-sixth of the eye is on show to the world. The rest sits cushioned in a bed of fat in the deep, bony eye socket. The eyeball itself is round, filled with a fluid-like gel that enables it to keep its shape. The wall of the eyeball has several layers. The outer one, called the sclera, or the "white" of the eye, is white and opaque. Just under this is a blood-rich layer known as the choroid, which supplies the eye with oxygen and nutrients.

The colour of your eyes is determined by which pigments are present in the iris. The iris is a circle, or diaphragm, of small muscles, which as they get bigger and smaller determine how much light is let in via the dark, black-looking opening called the pupil. The lens sits behind the pupil and focuses light onto the retina to give a clear and sharp picture.

eyebrows

The short hairs that make up our eyebrows help to give shape, definition, and expression to the face. If they are well-shaped, they can take years off your appearance by reducing the shadow cast over the eye and giving the illusion of lightening the whole face. Yet their role is not simply aesthetic. As well as framing the eyes, eyebrows are designed by nature to help create shade from sunlight and prevent perspiration dripping from the hairline and forehead into the eyes. Keeping them in good condition is as important for the health of the eye as it is for a sophisticated, sleek appearance.

eyelids

Like eyebrows, the eyelids are ideal areas for making-up in order to enhance and draw attention to your eyes. In addition, these very thin, skin-covered folds have a definite design function.The top eyelid is larger and much more mobile than the lower lid, and is able to raise and lower itself via its own supply of muscles. These muscles are "programmed" to blink around every three to seven seconds, and it is this involuntary action that helps to spread a thin film of salty, oily solution across the surface of the eyes, which prevents the eyes from drying out and the lids from sticking together. The solution is made and secreted from little ducts housed within the lids themselves. In addition to keeping the eyes moist, eyelids regulate how much light enters the eye and protect it from injury or irritation.

the conjunctiva

Lining the back surface of the eyelids is a very fine mucous membrane called the conjunctiva, the role of which is mainly to lubricate the eyes and stop them from drying out. Should this lining become inflamed or infected by bacteria, allergens, or even contact lenses, the resulting irritation is known as conjunctivitis.

tears

The inside of the eyelid is also where the tear glands are found. Continually releasing a dilute, salty, tear solution, tears certainly lubricate the eyes – but they do much more besides. Full of antibodies and bacteria-destroying enzymes, tears also cleanse and protect the eyes. When the eyes become irritated by grit or chemicals, or when we are upset, tear production increases. Because tears are known to contain natural opiates, it is thought that shedding tears may help to reduce stress when emotionally distraught, and even lessen pain when we are physically damaged.

Excess tears that are not wiped away disappear into two tiny holes on the side of the eyelids and through a series of tubes drain into the nose itself – which is why your nose runs when you cry.

eyelashes

The eyelashes grow from the edge of each eyelid. These fine hairs react the moment anything – even a puff of air – touches them, triggering a blink that protects the eye.

sinuses

The small, air-filled cavities within the skull, known as the sinuses, are designed to lighten the skull and give resonance to the voice. When inflamed and filled with mucus due to a cold-causing virus, bacterial infection, or allergens, the sinuses feel blocked and, due to their interconnections with the eyes, make the eyes water, redden, and run.

around the eyes

The delicate skin around the eyes is prone to fine lines and wrinkles. Everything from stress and fatigue to eyestrain and excess sun exposure can affect how many and how pronounced such lines can be.

beautiful eyes

You can help protect your eyes from environmental pollution and cleanse and care for them with a beauty regime. But just as with skin, hair, and nails, all parts of the eyes, including the lashes and eyebrows, rely on a balanced, constant supply of nutrients, water, and oxygen to remain in tip-top condition.

eye facts

- The eyes measure about 2.5cm (1 inch) across.
- Recent research suggests that certain plant nutrients may be able to help prevent diseases of the eye.
- In between the lashes are tiny glands. When these become blocked, infection can occur, which may lead to a stye.
- Betacarotene, the orange pigment found in carrots, mangoes, and peaches, is needed to help us see in the dark.
- Pilots flying in the Second World War reported better night vision when they were regularly eating blueberry jam.
- Recent research has indicated that the pigment lutein, found in yellow vegetables and fruits, may help reduce the risk of age-related blindness.
- Herbal teas, such as chamomile and goldenseal, may be used to bathe inflamed eyes. They can also be drunk to help relieve the same symptoms.
- Newborn babies do not produce tears for the first three months of life.

eye beauty foods

what apricots do

Apricots can help maintain **good vision** and keep the surface of the eye **moist**, **shining**, and free from dry, opaque spots, which interfere with sight. They can also be involved in reducing redness and keeping the skin of the eyelids in good condition, which lessens the chances of inflammation. Apricots can also give some **protection from the sun's** ultraviolet radiation.

why apricots work

Apricots supply the body with the orange pigment betacarotene, which is converted into vitamin A if supplies are running low. A lack of vitamin A can cause secretions in the eye to dry up, making the eyes red, swollen, painful, dry, and lustreless; this condition will eventually cause white spots and loss of vision. Betacarotene also acts as an antioxidant, helping protect the eye from sunlight and reducing the risk of damage to the lens proteins, which leads to cataracts.

apricot serving ideas

The stronger the colour of the apricot, the more betacarotene it contains and the sweeter the flavour. These fruits are delicious simply eaten raw. Alternatively, apricots can be poached with cardamom, stewed, made into crumbles, and added to flapjacks and stuffing. Ready-to-eat dried apricots make a tasty addition to a muesli mix, or they can be eaten as a healthy snack.

apricot watchpoints

Choose the darkest apricots available to maximize betacarotene intakes. Levels decrease slightly during the canning process.

apricots

for moist eyes and protection from the sun

Other eye-moistening foods

Carrots, kale, sweet potatoes, mangoes, peaches, eggs, liver

blueberries

improve the blood supply to the eyes

what blueberries do

Blueberries may help to keep the whites of the eyes **clear**, **bright**, and free from redness caused by the leaking of tiny broken capillaries. The small blueberry is used by medical herbalists to maintain **healthy vision** and help reduce problems with night-blindness. They may also reduce the risk of glaucoma as well as cataracts in later life.

why blueberries work

Blueberries are exceptionally rich in plant nutrients called flavonoids, particularly anthocyanidins, which strengthen collagen in the walls of the tiny blood vessels in the eyes, helping them dilate without breaks and bleeding. Bolstering capillary walls maintains a good supply of blood to the eye, which helps sustain pressure, preventing glaucoma. It also feeds protein structures in the lens, which, if starved, can become opaque and cause cataracts. Blueberries also supply vitamin C, another antioxidant vitamin that protects eye health.

blueberry serving ideas

Blueberries are wonderful eaten fresh, topped with plain fromage frais, and added to fruit salad or bowls of breakfast cereal. They can be dried and eaten as a snack, or added to breads and scones. The berries can also be stewed, used in stews, made into jam, or juiced. Extracts can be bought in supplement form.

blueberry watchpoints

When cooked or dried, the vitamin C in blueberries is lost, although the flavonoids remain intact. To get the most from them nutritionally, buy fresh, wash thoroughly, and eat within a few days.

Other blood vessel-strengthening foods

Cherries, grapes, strawberries, raspberries, green tea

Other free radical-fighting foods

Guavas, papayas, oranges, kiwi fruit, peppers, strawberries

spinach

neutralizes damaging free radicals

what spinach does

Spinach may help keep the eyes **clear**, **white**, and **glistening**, and the lids and tear ducts in good shape by fighting off infections. Regular servings of this green, leafy vegetable may also **protect** the lens of the eye from the sun's ultraviolet radiation, which can otherwise lead to blurred vision, squinting, and ultimately cataracts.

why spinach works

Vitamin C in spinach helps fight infections throughout the body. This may include infections in the eye that cause inflammation, redness of the eyelid linings, blocked tear ducts, and dryness. Spinach also contains betacarotene, which is normally associated with orange vegetables and fruits. Along with other carotenoids, this helps neutralize free radicals created by the sun's rays, and may reduce lens damage and the risk of cataracts.

spinach serving ideas

To get the most vitamin C from spinach, it is best to select baby leaves and eat them raw in a salad. Try the leaves mixed with dressing, lean, grilled bacon pieces, and crumbled blue cheese. Otherwise, lightly steam and cream with yoghurt, or serve as eggs Florentine. Spinach can be made into soup or gnocchi, or served in pasta dishes.

spinach watchpoints

Cooking spinach in large amounts of water leaches out vitamin C, although cooking does not destroy the carotenes. Avoid wilted, yellow, and damaged leaves, and store in the fridge to preserve the vitamin C content.

what yellow peppers do

Yellow peppers may help **reduce** the development of **fine lines** around the eyes by aiding the retention of **sharp vision**, which lessens the need to squint. They can also help to keep the eyes **moist** and **sparkly**, flush out grit and dust, and help fight off infections that lead to inflammation and redness.

why yellow peppers work

Yellow peppers, along with sweetcorn, spinach, bananas, and kale, are rich in the yellow pigment lutein (pronounced "loo-teen"). This antioxidant helps retain sharp vision by protecting the macula, the small central part of the retina that is responsible for central vision. When damaged, for example, by ultraviolet radiation due to exposure to the sun, the macula degenerates, eventually leading to blindness. Yellow peppers also supply vitamin C, which is needed to fight infections and keep the tear glands clear so that irritating particles can be safely washed away.

yellow pepper serving ideas

Sliced or chopped, yellow peppers can be eaten raw in salads, or used to top pizzas. Brushed with olive oil, they are excellent when grilled or roasted and served in salads. Yellow peppers can be made into soups, or used in dishes such as paella or ratatouille. Whole peppers can be cored, de-seeded, and stuffed with rice.

yellow pepper watchpoints

Avoid peppers with blemishes or wrinkles; their vitamin C levels will have plummeted. Wash well to remove pesticides before eating.

yellow peppers

protect the retina

Other retina-protecting foods

Bananas, star fruit, berries, mandarins, oranges, grapes, blackcurrants, sweetcorn

Other health-promoting foods

Sunflower seeds, sesame seeds, avocados, sweet potatoes, hazelnuts, almonds

wheat germ

promotes good eyelid health

what wheat germ does

Wheat germ can help to keep the **eyelids healthy**, both on their inside linings, so that the eyes do not appear puffy or swollen, and on their exterior, avoiding redness and soreness. Wheat germ may also help to ensure that the **blood vessels** of the eye are not become bloodshot.

why wheat germ works

Wheat germ is rich in vitamin E which keeps many tissue linings, including those inside the eyelids, in good condition. This can help avoid infections. It also supplies zinc, a mineral found in one of its highest concentrations in the eye; zinc works with vitamin C to resist infections and speed healing. Wheat germ also contains good amounts of iron, needed to ensure that plenty of oxygen reaches the eye so that vessels do not become bloodshot.

wheat germ serving ideas

Wheat germ can be sprinkled over breakfast cereals or stirred into yoghurt to give it a nutty flavour and extra volume. These small, creamy-looking flakes are also ideal for adding to bread and crumble mixes, and can be used to increase the nutritional value of fruit-smoothie drinks. Put a spoonful into stews and soups to boost your vitamins.

**Other infection-
fighting foods**
Garlic, leeks, strawberries,
green tea

echinacea

boosts the immune system

what echinacea does

Echinacea has been used by Native Americans for centuries to **boost** the **immune** system. If you are prone to styes, then taking extracts of this herb may help reduce their incidence at times of stress, as well as helping to heal those that have already developed. Echinacea can also play a role in keeping the eyes **bright**, **healthy**, and free from soreness, congestion, and redness.

why echinacea works

Echinacea is well-known for its ability to strengthen the immune system, making the body less susceptible to stress and so possibly reduce the development of styes. It also has specific abilities to ward off infections with its antibiotic properties. Capable, too, of improving the body's own production of interferon, echinacea is well-placed to join the fight against viral infections such as colds and flu, typical symptoms of which include tired, dull, watery eyes.

echinacea serving ideas

Ready-to-use tinctures and supplements are the most easily available way to take echinacea. The standardized dosage for tinctures is fifteen drops in a small amount of water three times a day.

echinacea watchpoints

The tincture can taste bitter and make the lips and tongue tingle, in which case supplements are advised. If allergic to any flower in the daisy family, check with your doctor before using. Take echinacea at the first sign of any infectious illness, but do not use for more than two to three weeks.

what brown rice does

The chances of having eyes **free from** tiny **broken** or engorged **capillaries** may be improved through regularly eating brown rice and other wholegrain cereals rich in fibre, especially when combined with plenty of water. These foods may also help the body to **deal better** with **stress** and tension, helping to keep the development of lines and crow's feet at bay.

why brown rice works

Brown rice and other fibrous cereal foods combine with water in the colon to create soft, bulky stools, which helps avoid constipation. Constipation and the straining associated with it increase blood pressure throughout the body, including in the eyes. This can lead to an increase in capillary size and small breaks and leaks that cause the eyes to become bloodshot. Brown rice also supplies the body with a range of B vitamins needed for handling stress.

brown rice serving ideas

Brown rice, with its slightly nutty flavour, can be used in place of white rice in many dishes. It can be used to stuff peppers or vine leaves, be added to soup, served in rice and peas, or with chillies, curries, or spicy lamb dishes. Cold rice makes an excellent base for a wide variety of filling salads, teaming up well with everything from seafood to apple and walnuts.

brown rice watchpoints

Brown rice takes longer to boil or steam than white rice, because the water has to penetrate its bran layers. Buy from reputable outlets to make sure the rice is free from any type of infestation.

brown rice

protects blood vessels

Other blood vessel-strengthening foods

Wholemeal bread, wholegrain breakfast cereals, brown pasta, oats

what grape-seed extract does

Grape-seed extract may help **relieve tension** and strain in the eyes after close work such as reading and computing. Reducing strain keeps the eyes looking **brighter** and can **reduce squinting**. Both by this effect and by directly preserving collagen, grape-seed extract may reduce the development of the fine lines and wrinkles in the skin around the eyes. It may also help retain **clear vision** in later life.

why grape-seed extract works

Grape-seed extract contains proanthocyanidins, substances that have a potent effect on tiny blood vessels throughout the body, including those in the eyes. Here, they may improve circulation and thus the supply of both oxygen and nutrients. Proanthocyanidins also strengthen capillary walls, possibly helping to stop eyes becoming bloodshot. Research shows that grape-seed extract improves eyestrain and thus may also help lower the chances of lens damage, cataracts, and loss of sight through damage to the retina.

grape-seed extract serving ideas

Grape-seed extract can be taken only in supplement form and is available as a powdered version in capsules, in a liquid form, or as a tablet. Pycnogenols, which also contain proanthocyanidins, are similar substances available ino an extract; they come from the Mediterranean pine rather than grape seeds. For general protection of the eyes, take 100mg daily.

grape-seed extract watchpoints

Proanthocyanidins remain active in the body only for a limited time, so to get the full benefit of their health-giving properties, it is best to take supplements regularly at breakfast, lunch, and dinner.

grape-seed extract

relieves eye tension

Other tension-relieving foods

Blueberries, grapes, cherries, oranges, green tea

Other sleep-enhancing foods

Milk, yoghurt, fromage frais, bananas, kava kava, St John's wort

chamomile

reduces dark circles

what chamomile does

Chamomile can play a part in **improving** the look of dull, tired eyes and helping **reduce dark circles** and "bags" in the skin beneath. This well-known herb may play a role in reducing the formation of **fine lines** and crow's feet in the area around the eyes. Chamomile can also help keep the eyes **moist**, **bright**, and free from redness and soreness.

why chamomile works

Valerianic acid in the leaves of the chamomile plant encourages a good night's sleep, and so may help reduce the appearance of dark circles under the eyes. By soothing nerves and promoting relaxation, facial tension around the eyes is relieved, potentially helping to reduce the formation of wrinkles. Known for its antiseptic properties, chamomile may help the body fight infections on the inside linings of the eyelid which otherwise lead to inflammation, redness, and blocked tear ducts.

chamomile serving ideas

A tea can be made from the dried flowers by adding 500ml (18fl oz) of water to 25g (1oz) of herbs and steeping for ten minutes. The tea can be drunk hot with a little honey during the day and before bedtime. Chamomile tincture can be taken or five to ten drops can be added to warm water and used as an eyewash. Capsules are also available.

chamomile watchpoints

Chamomile stimulates the uterus and thus should be avoided during pregnancy. It is wise to stick to the suggested intake with supplements, or two to three cups of tea daily.

eye
beauty diet

Gritty, blurry, dry eyes not only make you feel unattractive, they are also distressing. The right diet can help combat such passing symptoms, while lifelong attention to diet may lower your chances of contracting cataracts, glaucoma, and macular degeneration, all of which impair vision.

The following diet is rich in essential fats found in oily fish, nuts, and seeds, to help reduce eye dryness, while vitamin E in wheat germ may protect the lining of the eye from the effects of pollution and tobacco smoke. Betacarotene in apricots and spinach is converted into vitamin A, which is needed to keep eye tissue moist and lubricated, and to protect against ultraviolet radiation. New research is revealing how another carotene, called lutein, which is found in yellow peppers and sweetcorn, can act to prevent loss of sight. Anthocyanidins in blueberries may help reduce bloodshot eyes, while vitamin C in the fruits and vegetables used will boost resistance to infections such as colds and conjunctivitis – both renowned for clouding vision and making the eyes stream.

5–day clear-eye diet

	breakfast	**lunch**	**dinner**
1	peach and wheat germ shake	yellow pepper soup	curried salad with spiced tofu
2	blueberry bran flakes	pasta and prawn salad with three-mustard tomato dressing	grilled cod with a herb crust
3	orange and cardamom baked bananas	tagliatelle with spinach, pine nuts, and raisins	sweet potato and fish skewers
4	apricot and peach fruit salad	celeriac and almond soup	aromatic salmon
5	blueberry and oatmeal yoghurt	sweetcorn chowder	warm seafood salad

day 1 *recipes*

peach and wheat germ shake

1 ripe peach, stoned
150ml (5fl oz) milk or soya milk
1 tbsp wheat germ
1 tsp honey
crushed ice, to serve

1. Blend all ingredients together until smooth.
2. Pour into a chilled glass over crushed ice and serve immediately.

yellow pepper soup

225ml (8fl oz) vegetable stock (use an organic stock cube)
1 yellow pepper, de-seeded and chopped
1 potato, peeled and chopped
2 carrots, peeled and chopped
salt and freshly ground black pepper

1. Put the vegetable stock in a pan and add the pepper, potato, carrots, and seasoning. Simmer for twenty minutes, or until the vegetables are tender.
2. Cool the soup slightly, then purée in a blender or food processor. Return to the pan and heat through.
3. Adjust the seasoning, then serve with granary bread.

curried salad with spiced tofu

100g (3½oz) plain tofu
salt and freshly ground black pepper
pinch of cayenne pepper, paprika, and curry powder
1 tbsp mango chutney
1 tbsp sultanas, soaked in hot water
juice of ½ lemon
4 sprigs curly parsley, finely chopped
4 heaped tbsp cooked rice
1 red pepper
½ cucumber, de-seeded and peeled
salad leaves and tomatoes, to serve

1. Pre-heat the grill to maximum.
2. Place the tofu on a baking tray, season with a pinch of salt and the spices, and grill for five to six minutes, turning halfway through. Remove and cut into chunks.
3. Place the mango chutney in a bowl with the soaked sultanas, lemon juice, and freshly chopped parsley. Add the cooked rice; season lightly.
4. De-seed, then dice the pepper and cucumber and add to the rice salad. Mix half the tofu with the salad and add the rest on top. Serve with salad leaves and sliced tomatoes.

day 2 *recipes*

blueberry bran flakes

40g (½1oz) bran flakes

125ml (4fl oz) cold milk

50g (1¾oz) fresh blueberries

1. Pour the bran flakes into a bowl.
2. Pour on the chilled milk, and sprinkle with blueberries.

pasta and prawn salad with three-mustard tomato dressing

1 head broccoli, broken into florets

125g (4½oz) cooked wholegrain pasta

100g (3½oz) cooked, peeled prawns

1 small bunch flat-leaf parsley, chopped

For the dressing

3 very ripe tomatoes, skinned

1 tsp tomato purée

1 tsp each of Dijon, grain, and French mustard

2 tsp white wine vinegar

2 tsp granulated sugar

1 tbsp fat-free vinaigrette dressing

salt and freshly ground black pepper

1. Cook the broccoli in boiling water for three to four minutes.
2. Place all the ingredients for the dressing in a liquidizer or food processor and blend until smooth. It is important to make sure that the mustard and tomato dressing does not taste too sweet or too acidic. Season to your own taste, either with a little more sugar or a touch of vinegar.
3. Add the dressing to the cooked pasta and prawns, then stir in the cooked broccoli and chopped parsley. Serve either hot or cold.

grilled cod with a herb crust

2 slices wholemeal bread

1 tbsp chopped parsley

salt and freshly ground black pepper

juice of 1 lime

100g (3½oz) skinless cod fillet

100g (3½oz) green beans

100g (3½oz) baby carrots

1 tbsp fat-free salad dressing

1. Pre-heat oven to 200°C/400°F/gas mark 6–7.
2. In a food processor or blender, grind the wholemeal bread into crumbs. Add the chopped parsley with a little salt and pepper, and continue to blend until the crumbs turn slightly green.
3. Squeeze the lime juice over the cod and season. Pack the herb crumbs over the cod fillet on one side only, place on a baking tray, and bake until the herb crust starts to turn golden brown – around seven to eight minutes.
4. Meanwhile, cook the vegetables either by steaming or microwaving with a little water. Drain, then mix together with the salad dressing. Once the fish is ready, serve on the bed of vegetables and spoon over any remaining cooking juices.

day 3 *recipes*

orange and cardamom baked bananas

vanilla essence

1 tbsp orange juice

1 tsp brown sugar

freshly crushed cardamom seeds

1 large banana, peeled

2 tbsp plain fromage frais

1. Cut an oval of foil large enough to fit the banana. Sprinkle a little vanilla essence, the orange juice, brown sugar, and a few cardamom seeds onto the foil, then add the banana.
2. Fold up the foil and bake in a hot oven for five minutes. Serve some fromage frais.

tagliatelle with spinach, pine nuts, and raisins

375g (13oz) fresh young spinach leaves

85g (3oz) wholegrain tagliatelle

1 tsp extra-virgin olive oil

1 tbsp pine nuts

1 tsp raisins

salt and freshly ground black pepper

freshly grated nutmeg

1. Rinse the spinach and discard any tough stalks. Put into a large pan using just the water that remains on the leaves. Cover and cook on a medium heat, tossing occasionally, until just wilted. Drain and squeeze out as much water as possible.
2. Cook the tagliatelle in plenty of boiling salted water until *al dente* and drain well.
3. Coat a frying pan lightly with the oil and heat. Add the pine nuts and raisins, and fry for a couple of minutes, then add the spinach and season with salt, black pepper, and nutmeg to taste.
4. Toss over the heat until warmed through, then serve immediately with the tagliatelle.

sweet potato and fish skewers

1 large sweet potato, cooked in its jacket

85g (3oz) white fish, cut into large chunks

6 button mushrooms

2 tsp runny honey

2 tsp grain mustard

2 tsp soy sauce

2 carrots, peeled

juice of half a lemon

1 tsp sugar

1. Pre-heat grill to maximum. Cut the sweet potato into six large chunks, then thread them onto two skewers, alternating with chunks of white fish and mushrooms.
2. Mix together the honey, mustard, and soy sauce, and brush onto the skewers. Place on a suitable baking tray and then grill for four to five minutes, turning once halfway through the cooking time.
3. Meanwhile, finely grate the carrots, mix with the lemon juice, and season with a little salt and the sugar.
4. Serve the potato skewers with the carrot salad.

day 4 *recipes*

apricot and peach fruit salad

1 dried fig
2 dried prunes
2 dried apricots
1 dried peach half
1 dried pear half
1 dried apple ring
1 clove
50ml (2oz) water
1 tsp honey (optional)
1 tbsp plain fromage frais
1 tsp chopped pumpkin seeds

1. Wash the fruit and put in a pan with the clove and water to soak overnight.
2. In the morning, bring the water to the boil and simmer the fruit for twenty minutes, adding more water if necessary.
3. Add the honey, if necessary to sweeten, and serve warm topped with the fromage frais and scattered with the pumpkin seeds.

aromatic salmon

85g (3oz) salmon fillet
1 lemon grass blade, finely chopped
1cm (½ inch) piece fresh ginger, grated
grated zest of 1 lemon
150g (5½oz) fresh egg noodles
sunflower oil
85g (3oz) fresh bean sprouts
½ tsp fish sauce
½ tsp soy sauce

1. Place the salmon in a steamer with the lemon grass, ginger, and lemon zest and steam for six minutes.
2. Meanwhile, cook the noodles according to the packet instructions.
3. Heat the oil and quickly sauté the fresh bean sprouts with the fish and soy sauce.
4. Drain and serve the noodles with the bean sprouts and salmon.

celeriac and almond soup

2 tsp flaked almonds
extra-virgin olive oil
1 shallot or small onion, peeled and chopped
½ small celeriac, peeled and sliced
225ml (8fl oz) vegetable stock (use an organic stock cube)
2 tbsp plain yoghurt
freshly ground black pepper

1. Toast the almonds under a grill for a few minutes until golden. Reserve a few for garnish; finely grind the rest.
2. Brush a pan lightly with olive oil and gently cook the onion until soft. Add the celeriac and stock, and bring to the boil. Cover and simmer for thirty minutes, or until the celeriac is tender. Transfer to a blender; purée till smooth.
3. Return the soup to the pan, stir in the yoghurt and ground almonds, and gently re-heat. Season with pepper, garnish with the reserved flaked almonds, and serve with a wholemeal roll.

day 5 *recipes*

blueberry and oatmeal yoghurt

1 tbsp toasted oatmeal

100g (3½oz) blueberries

150g (5½oz) bio-yoghurt or soya yoghurt

1 tsp honey-roast sunflower seeds

1. Stir the oatmeal and half the blueberries into the yoghurt.
2. Scatter with the remaining blueberries and sunflower seeds and serve.

sweetcorn chowder

50g (1¾oz) cooked turkey breast

extra-virgin olive oil

1 leek, thinly sliced

200ml (7fl oz) chicken stock (use an organic stock cube)

1 small can sweetcorn

freshly ground black pepper

warm wholegrain pitta bread, to serve

1. Slice the turkey into strips.
2. Brush a pan lightly with the oil and gently cook the leeks until transparent, then add the turkey strips to warm through.
3. Put half the stock into a food processor and blend with half the sweetcorn. Add the remaining stock, blend, then stir in with the leek and turkey.
4. Heat until piping hot, season with black pepper, and serve with warm pitta bread.

warm seafood salad

selection of salad leaves: lollo rosso, radicchio, frisé

1 tsp extra-virgin olive oil

½ tsp tarragon vinegar

1 tsp chopped tarragon

salt and freshly ground black pepper

60g (2¼oz) asparagus, trimmed

60g (2¼oz) lemon sole fillet, skinned

4 tsp white wine

25g (1oz) scallops or peeled prawns

chunk of fresh bread, to serve

1. Arrange the salad leaves on a plate. Mix together the oil, vinegar, tarragon, and seasoning to make a dressing and set aside.
2. Steam the asparagus for seven minutes, until tender. While it is cooking, cut the fish fillet in half lengthways, then across into thin strips. Place the fish and the wine in a frying pan and simmer until almost cooked. Add the scallops or prawns and cook for a further two minutes.
3. Lift fish from the pan and put onto the salad leaves, then top with the asparagus. Pour on the dressing and serve with a chunk of fresh bread.

eye
beauty massage

Nowhere does tiredness show more than in the eyes. Completing this carefully developed set of massages can help stimulate circulation and ensure a good flow of rejuvenating oxygen and nutrients to the eyes, restoring the sparkle while also helping to comfort and soothe. Two of the massages also reveal how gentle, carefully applied pressure to specific points can help tackle and clear blocked sinuses and reduce puffiness. Designed to release stress around the eyes, completing the eye massages at least once a week may also help to keep fine lines at bay.

stimulate circulation around the eyes

1 Use your ring fingers, which have the lightest touch, to circle your eyes. Start firmly at the centre of the eyebrows and stroke along the eyebrows, gliding gently back under the eyes.

2 Keep the pressure extremely light below the eyes and be careful not to stretch the skin. Repeat the movement five times.

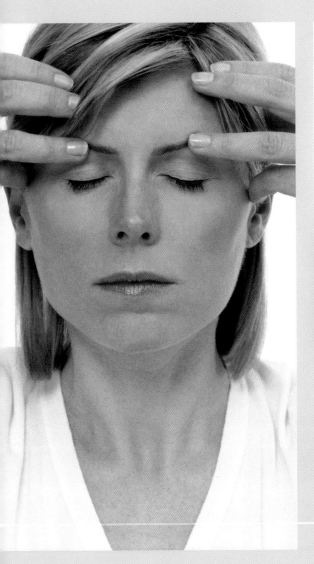

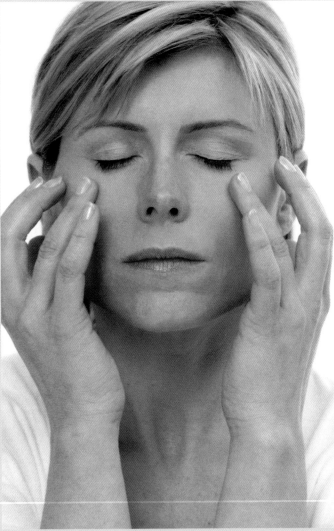

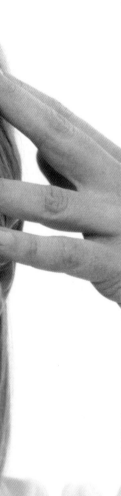

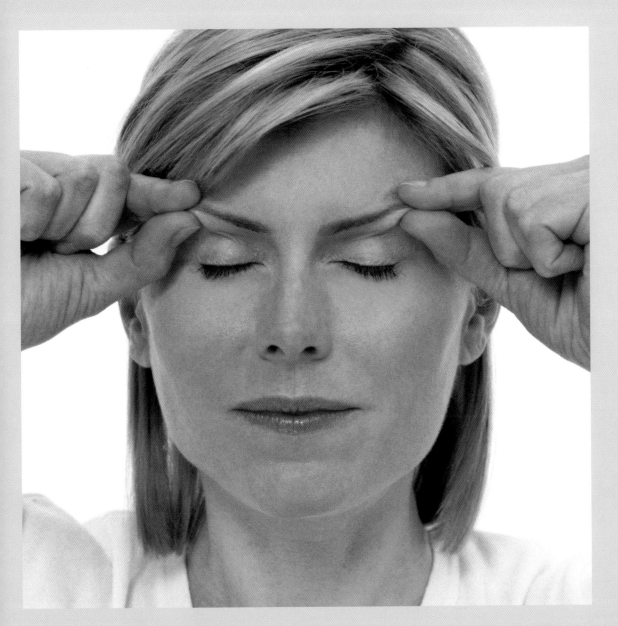

awaken the eyes

Using your thumbs and index fingers, start at the bridge of the nose between the eyes and pinch gently but firmly along each eyebrow. Hold each pinch for a few seconds, then release and squeeze a little further along. Continue this action out toward the temples. Repeat three times.

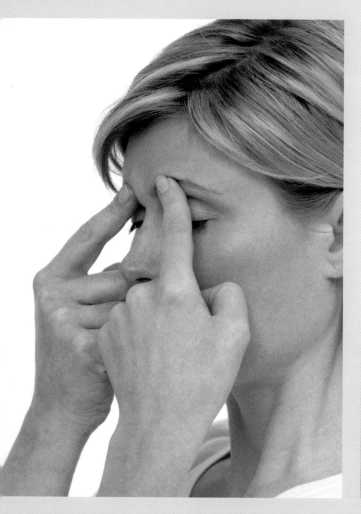

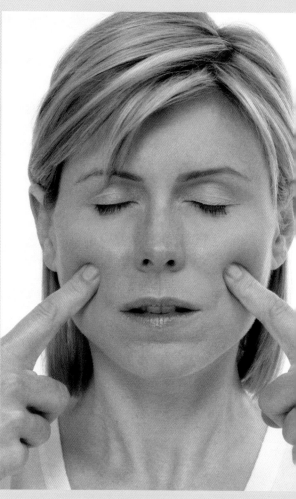

clear sinuses and reduce puffiness

Using your index fingers, apply pressure to each eye, starting at the bridge of the nose, just below your eyebrows. Hold for a couple of seconds, then release. Move to the base of the nose (where it meets your cheek), apply firm pressure for a couple of seconds, then release.

Slide your finger along the bottom of your cheekbones, level with the middle of your eyes, until you find two small indentations in the bone. Hold for a couple of seconds, then release. Repeat three times.

restore sparkle to the eyes

Using the tips of your fingers, tap extremely lightly all the way around your eyes, then over the closed eyelids. The action should be like a butterfly gently flapping its wings. Do this for approximately thirty seconds.

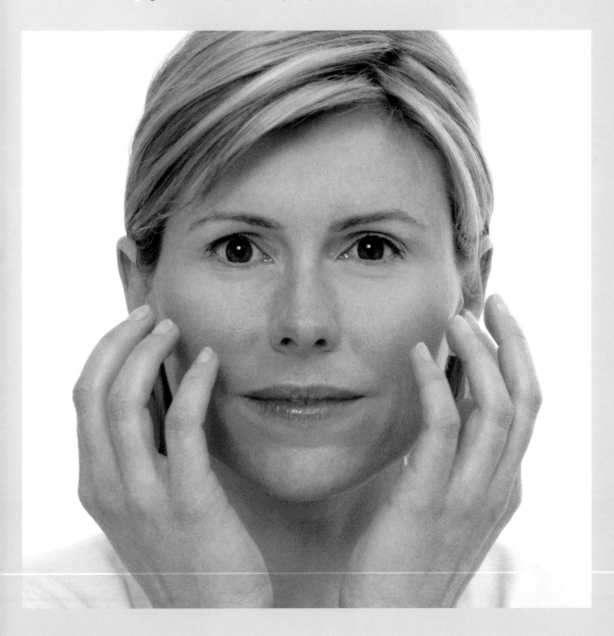

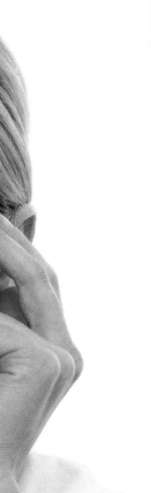

2 Now repeat the exercise with your left hand over your left eye.

Note: These two movements can be combined using both hands at the same time.

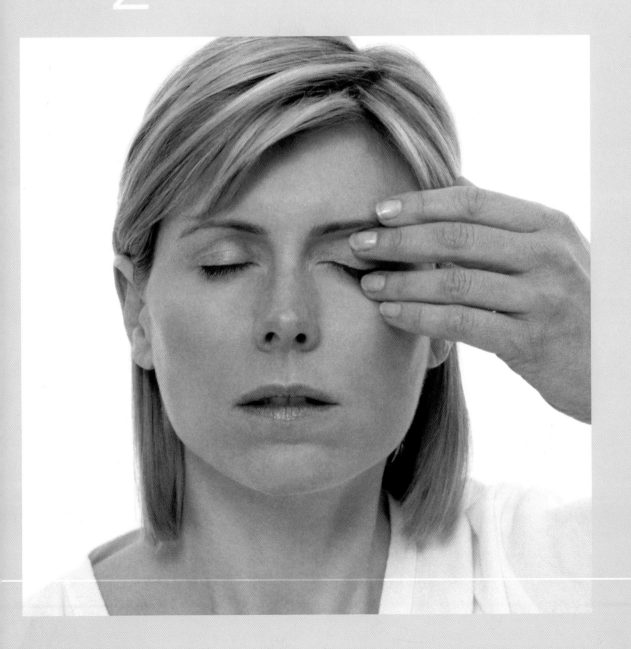

beauty foods
pharmacy

skin problem	which food	why
acne	sweet potatoes, carrots, kale, mangoes, peaches	supply betacarotene, which is converted into vitamin A. Vitamin A may reduce symptoms
	bananas, lettuce, kava kava, valerian tea, chamomile tea	reduce stress, which increases the risk of acne
	oysters, pine nuts, sesame seeds, cashew nuts	rich in zinc, which is needed for wound healing
broken thread veins	wholegrain cereals, water	reduce constipation and blood pressure
	berries, grapes, green tea, grape-seed extract	strengthen blood vessel walls
eczema	evening primrose oil, blackcurrant oil, sunflower and sesame seeds	increase the production of prostaglandins, which reduce itching, and inflammation
	grape-seed extract	reduce the allergic reaction
	oysters and wholegrain cereals	promote healing of injured skin
hives	anise, ginger and peppermint teas	antihistamine effects reduce allergic responses
	apples, onions, grapes, tea	contain quercetin, which stops histamine release
	valerian tea, kava kava	reduce stress, which can trigger hives
psoriasis	mackerel, sardines, tuna, salmon, flax seeds, Brazil nuts	supply omega-3 essential fats and selenium that dampen inflammatory processes
	wheat germ	rich in vitamin E for healing damaged skin
spots	water and dandelion, nettle and burdock tea	stimulate the kidneys, detoxify the system and purify the blood. Burdock also has antibiotic effects
	evening primrose oil, Agnus castus	balance hormonal changes that trigger spots
sunburn	water, watermelon, cucumber	rehydrate the skin
	carrots, sweet potatoes, mangoes, peppers, guava, citrus fruits, wheat germ, nuts, seeds	supply betacarotene and vitamins C and E to reduce free radicals from excess UV radiation
thinning skin	soya beans/ milk/yoghurt, tofu, flax seeds	contain plant oestrogens, which may boost collagen synthesis, and reduce thinning

skin problem	which food	why
wrinkles and frown lines	horsetail tea, oats, museli, berries, glucosamine	improve the structure and growth of collagen and elastin, repair damage, boost circulation
	chamomile tea, st John's wort	reduce stress and frowning

nail problem	which food	why
brittle nails	horsetail tea, oat-straw tea, oats, muesli	supply silica, used by therapists to help improve thickness and strength of the nails
infections	garlic, onions, leeks, spring onions	contain allicin, a plant nutrient with antifungal properties which helps fight infections
thinning nails	eggs	supply the B vitamin biotin, needed for the development of keratin, the hard nail protein
vertical ridges	oily fish, red meat, dark poultry, fortified breakfast cereals, cashew nuts, sesame seeds	rich in iron, a lack of which causes anaemia, for which ridged nails are a symptom
white flecks	oysters, fortified breakfast cereals, pine nuts, sesame seeds and cashew nuts	provide the mineral zinc, a lack of which is associated with white marks on the nail

mouth problem	which food	why
bad breath	parsley	contains chlorophyll, which combats odours
	xylitol-sweetened chewing gum	helps kill bacteria that can cause bad breath
	aniseed, cardamom, caraway seeds, coriander, fennel seeds	help freshen the breath after eating
	water	for maximum saliva to wash away bacteria
bleeding gums	green tea	helps fight gum disease with flavanols
	berries	rich in anthocyanins, which strengthen blood-vessel walls
cold sores	chicken, fish, pulses, eggs, meat, brewers' yeast	rich in the protein lysine, which directly reduces the activity of the cold-sore-causing herpes simplex virus
cracked lips	mackerel, soya beans, almonds, cottage cheese, fortified breakfast cereals, milk, yoghurt	rich in riboflavin (vitamin B_2), a lack of which causes swollen, cracked lips and fissures at the corners of the lips
mouth ulcers	onions, spring onions	natural antiseptic properties to help heal infections in the ulcers
	apples, grapes, onions	supply quercetin, which reduces inflammation

mouth problem	which food	why
mouth ulcers continued	guava, peppers, berries, spinach	heal damaged cheek cells
swollen tongue	sesame and sunflower seeds, fortified breakfast cereals, black-eyed peas, citrus fruit, fish, poultry, eggs	supply iron, vitamins B_2 and B_{12} and folic acid, all of which contribute to a healthy tongue
tooth decay	cheese	supplies the protein casein which helps enamel repair itself. Also lowers mouth acidity and supplies calcium for strong enamel
	xylitol-sweetened chewing gum	reduces activity of the decay-causing bacteria, fights plaque and lowers acidity of the mouth, all of which protect against decay

hair problem	which food	why
brittle hair	oat-straw tea, horsetail tea (or supplements), oats, muesli	contain silica, shown in some trials to reduce brittleness after several months of use
flaky scalp	salmon, mackerel, tuna, flax seeds, evening primrose oil, sunflower and sesame seeds	provide omega-3 and -6 fatty acids needed for a well-hydrated, moisturized scalp
greying	crab, sunflower seeds, cashew nuts, almonds	supply copper, which is needed for the formation of hair pigments
hair loss	lettuce, bananas, valerian, kava kava	help reduce stress levels, a side-effect of which can be alopecia, or patchy hair loss
lifeless, dull hair	probiotic yoghurts and yoghurt drinks	supply "good bacteria" to improve nutrient digestion and fight infections
	wheat, bananas, oats, leeks, onions, Jerusalem artichokes, chicory root	help foster probiotic, or good, bacteria
slow growth	haddock, seaweed, mullet, mussels, whiting, cod	provide iodine for the production of the thyroid hormone thyroxin, a lack of which slows growth
thinning hair	red meat, oily fish, dark poultry meat, sesame and sunflower seeds, fortified breakfast cereals, pulses	all supply iron, a lack of which leads to sub-clinical and full-blown anaemia, both of which can result in thinning of the hair

eye problem	which food	why
bloodshot eyes	wholegrain cereals, wholemeal bread, brown rice and brown pasta, water	reduce the risk of constipation. Straining can increase pressure in the eye and lead to engorged and broken blood vessels
	berries, green tea, grape-seed extract	contain blood-vessel-strengthening plant nutrients to help prevent leakage
conjunctivitis	ju hua tincture	antibacterial and anti-inflammatory effects
	red meat, oysters, pine nuts, sesame and sunflower seeds	rich in zinc, which is needed to bolster the immune system and ward off infections
	wheat germ, avocado, dark-green leafy vegetables, peanuts, pinenuts, sunflower seeds	supply vitamin E needed for the health of the conjunctiva lining of the eyelid
dark circles	chamomile tea, lettuce, gotu kola, passion-flower	encourage a good night's sleep
dry, gritty eyes	evening primrose oil	shown in research to improve tear production and dry eyes in Sjögren's syndrome
	carrots, sweet potatoes, kale, mangoes	supply betacarotene, which is converted into vitamin A, needed for healthy tear ducts. A severe lack of vitamin A leads to xeropthalmia, which causes very dry eyes
hayfever	apples, onions, grapes, grape-seed extract, green tea	contain quercetin, which stops histamine release
	nettle tea	combined with quercetin-rich foods, this can reduce inflammation in the nose and help reduce itching and sneezing
	anise, ginger and peppermint teas	all have an antihistamine effects
	garlic	helps reduce allergic reactions
sinusitis	probiotic yoghurts	replace good bacteria to help fight infection
	green tea, grapes, apples, onions, grape-seed extract	contain quercetin, which stops histamine release
	oily fish, flax seeds	contain omega-3 fatty acids, which reduce inflammation
styes	carrots, sweet potatoes, kale, spinach, mangoes	provide betacarotene, needed to keep oil ducts free from blockages and infections
	probiotic yoghurts and yoghurt drinks	provide probiotic bacteria, which help boost the immune system, making the body less prone to infection

glossary

allicin: Broad-spectrum antibiotic substance found in garlic. Allicin is broken down into other compounds which have a range of therapeutic effects, including antiviral, antibacterial, and antifungal. Onions, spring onions, leeks, and shallots contain small amounts of allicin.

alopecia: Another name for baldness. Alopecia areata is a patchy baldness that is often temporary and is thought to be caused by shock or anxiety.

amalgam: Silver-looking dental filling used to fill decayed teeth, which contains mercury, silver, and tin.

antibiotics: Drugs designed to fight bacterial infections in the body. Antibiotics adversely affect the beneficial bacteria that live in the gut. Probiotic foods should be taken at the same time to help restore the balance and boost the immune system.

antioxidant: Substance that inhibits oxidation. Antioxidants are thought to protect cells from attack by free radicals. Vitamins C and E, many plant pigments such as betacarotene and lutein, and the minerals selenium and zinc have antioxidant qualities.

cataract: Opaque covering of the lens of the eye, which blurs vision and eventually leads to blindness.

coenzyme Q_{10}: Also known as Co-Q_{10}. A powerful antioxidant present in every cell in the body. It is crucial for energy production and has helps cure gum disease.

collagen: Bundles of spongy protein fibres present in skin, muscles, and tendons. The dermis is 95 per cent collagen, giving the skin structure and the ability to absorb shock.

dehydration: Occurs when fluid loss is not met by fluid replacement. Adversely affects the texture and appearance of the skin, eyes, nails, mouth, and hair.

dermis: Layer of skin that houses blood supply, hair roots and follicles, sweat glands.

echinacea: Herb native to North America that has antibiotic, immune-boosting, and anti-allergic effects in the body.

elastin: Stretchy type of protein found in the dermis of the skin, which gives the skin its elasticity.

EPA: Eicosapentanoic acid. A fatty acid found in oily fish, which, when broken down in the body, is made into anti-inflammatory types of prostaglandins.

epidermis: Layer of the skin that creates the top, waterproof, visible covering of the skin which is composed of dead cells.

free radicals: Naturally-occurring oxygen molecules that attack cell membranes. Free-radical damage is increased by exposure to the sun, pollution, and alcohol. Free radicals attack skin cells and increase production of MMP-1 enzyme (*see* below). It is thought that excess free radicals can be "mopped up" and deactivated by antioxidants.

GLA: Gamma linolenic acid. Fatty acid found in evening primrose and blackcurrant oil that is converted into the types of prostaglandins that help reduce inflammation and appear to help modulate hormone levels in the body.

glutathione: Powerful antioxidant that occurs widely in plant and animal tissues, including those of the human body.

haemoglobin: Red pigment in blood, made up of an iron-containing substance called "haem". Combines with and releases oxygen.

herpes simplex virus: The virus that causes cold sores. The herpes simplex virus can sit dormant in the nerve endings in the cheeks and, when stimulated (through stress, sun, or cold, for example) can become active, migrate to the lip margin and set up a cold-sore infection.

interferon: Protein made in body cells that prevents duplication of some infectious viruses.

isoflavones: Plant nutrients in soya-based foods and legumes that seem to mimic the effect of human oestrogen in the body.

lignins: Plant nutrients thought to have oestrogen-like effects. Present in flax seeds, rye bread bran, sesame seeds, some nuts.

lutein: Pronounced "loo-teen". A yellow/orange pigment found in foods such as yellow peppers, sweetcorn, and bananas, which appears to be particularly effective at protecting the eye from free-radical damage.

lymph: The fluid contained in the lymphatic vessels. It is transparent, colourless, or slightly yellow. The lymph glands produce lymphocytes, a type of white blood cell that is involved in the body's immune system.

macular degeneration: Destruction of part of the retina in the eye, which eventually leads to blindness.

melanin: Pigment found in the skin, hair, and parts of the eye.

methionine: Sulphur-containing amino acid needed in the diet for the production of keratin, a protein found in the hair.

mmp-1: Enzyme released in the skin which breaks down collagen. Radiation and smoking both seem to increase its production.

nail bed: The well-nourished bed upon which the nail plate sits.

nail matrix: Area from which the nail grows.

oestrogen: Hormones produced by the ovaries that control the menstrual cycle and affect the condition of skin, nails, and hair.

pcos: Proanthocyanidins. Antioxidant pigments found in the bark, stems, leaves and skins of plants, including many fruits and vegetables.

prostaglandins: Hormone-like substances that control certain reactions in the body. Some play a role in inflammatory processes, while others modulate hormonal activity.

serotonin: Substance widely distributed in the body, but especially prevalent in the lining of the brain. Believed to help control moods and emotions. A lack of serotonin can lead to depression.

silicon: Trace element found in the skin, nails, and hair, believed to be important in their structure.

striations: Longitudinal ridges on the nails, thought by some to be caused by dietary deficiencies.

superoxide dismutase: An enzyme in the body that is also an important antioxidant.

tannin: Soluble, astringent substance found in plants, thought to have antioxidant effects, and decrease inflammation.

tincture: Herbal solution made by steeping dried or fresh herbs in alcohol and water.

ultraviolet a rays: Solar radiation that causes some sunburn but also penetrates to the dermis, where the rays stimulate collagenase and elastase, enzymes that break down collagen and elastin, and age the skin.

ultraviolet b rays: Solar radiation that penetrates and can cause damage to the upper layers of skin. UVB rays are known to damage the oils on the skin's surface, drying the skin. They also cause cells to become swollen and pink, the condition called sunburn. It is this damage to the cells which can lead to cancer of the skin. The damage also leads to the production of free radicals.

valepotriates: Active constituent in the herb valerian, which has calming effects on the body and helps in insomnia.

valerianic acid: Active constituent in the herb valerian. *See* valepotriates.

xylitol: Sugar alcohol derived from the birch tree; used to sweeten sugar-free gum; also naturally present in some foods such as yellow plums. Reduces growth in the mouth of the *Streptococcus mutans* bacterium, increases saliva flow, and lowers acidity.

useful addresses

British Dietetic Association

Advice on how to find a State Registered Dietitian for one to one dietetic advice.
5th Floor, Charles House, 148/9 Great Charles Street, Birmingham, B3 3HT
Tel 0121 200 8080

British Academy of Aesthetic Dentists

Lists qualified dentists able to carry out restorative work with an aesthetic basis.
Suite 152, 84 Marylebone High Street, London, W1M 3DE
Tel 020 7636 9933

British Massage Therapy Council

For a list of local massage therapists.
Greenbank House, 65a Adelphi Street, Preston, PR1 7BH
Tel 01772 881063

British Society of Dermatologists

For finding a registered dermatologists. They only accept telephone calls.
Tel 020 7383 0266

National Institute for Medical Herbalists

Provides a list of qualified medical herbalists to find local practitioner.
56 Longbrook Street, Exeter, EX4 6AH
Tel 01392 426022

The Institute of Trichologists

Advice on members for expert help with hair problems.
Stockwell Road, London, SW9 9SU
Tel 08706 070602

International Stress Management Association (UK)

Write in for information on your nearest practitioner.
Southbank University, LPSS, 103 Borough Road, London, SE1 OAA

The Society of Chiropodists and Podiatrists

For information of nearest practitioners.
53 Welbeck Street, London, W1M 7HE
Tel 020 7234 8620

acknowledgements

My very special thanks to Annie O'Dell. Annie is a qualified professional massage therapist who designed the wonderful facial massages. She runs a private practice, teaches at the Clare Maxwell-Hudson Centre, works at St George's Hospital in London, and still manages to look calm! A huge thank you as ever to Peter Vaughan for your scrummy recipes and to Mike Prior for your time and effort on the cover shot. Finally a massive thank you to Becca, Nicky, Jamie A and Jamie G at Mitchell Beazley and to Russell for the fabby food and massage shots.

Mitchell Beazley would like to thank Ocean Spray for supplying cranberries for the photograph featured on page 54.

index

Page numbers in bold indicate a
main entry